JAIKRISHNADAS AYURVEDA SERIES
383

Epigenetics and Ayurveda

By
Dr. Pooja Sabharwal
(BAMS, MD, PHD, PGDHM, PGDYOGA, PGDAST, CFN)

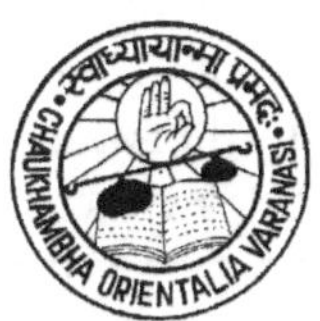

CHAUKHAMBHA ORIENTALIA
A House of Oriental, Antiquarian and Ayurvedic Books
VARANASI | BANGALORE

Epigenetics and Ayurveda

Pages : 124

© **Chaukhambha Orientalia**

First Edition : 2021
Digital Edition : 2024

Publishers :

CHAUKHAMBHA ORIENTALIA
Gokul Bhawan, K. 37/109,
Gopal Mandir Lane, Golghar, Maidagin
Varanasi-221001 (U.P.) (India)
Phone: 0542-2333476, 2334356
E-mail: co@chaukhambha.com ● info.covns@gmail.com

Branch : Poonam Plaza,
1ˢᵗ floor, No. 2602, 26ᵗʰ Main,
38ᵗʰ Cross, 9ᵗʰ Block, Jayanagar
Bangalore-560041
Phone: 080-43772098, 08105740600
E-mail: info.coktk@gmail.com
Website: www.chaukhambha.com

Disclaimer: The writers have tried their best in giving information available to them while preparing the material for this book. It is possible some errors might have been left uncorrected. The publisher and the writers will not be held any responsiblty for the errors, omissions or inaccuracies.

Digitalized by: Chaukhambha Orientalia (for KDP)

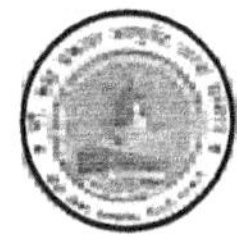

Ch. Brahm Prakash Ayurved Charak Sansthan
[Under Govt. of N.C.T. of Delhi]
Khera Dabar, Najafgath, New Delhi-110073

FOREWORD

It is really a privilege to write the foreword for the book entitled **'Epigenetics & Ayurveda'**. by a young authoress Dr. Pooja Sabharwal. There is a explicit demand of scientific understanding of fundamental concepts of Ayurveda worldwide. It is is also rightly advocated by Government of India through Niti Aayog to generate scientific evidences to prove basic ideologies of Ayurveda.

Holistic biology of *Ayurveda* is based on *Triguna, Tanmatra, Tridosha, Saptdhatu, Oja, Agni, Ama* and *Srotas.* *Srotas* are the inner transport system of the body which provide platform to carry out the structural, functional and psychological activities of other important bio factors like *Oja, Agni, Dhatu* etc. According to Ayurveda, treatment of the disease is not only to cure the symptoms but brings the person back to his her true nature. Ayurveda works to make the body disease free by its complete annihilation along with its root causes. This Epigenetic research confirms that traditional ancient knowledge of diet, lifestyle and mindfulness can all be used to fight disease and promote health. We are here on this planet to optimize the expression of our genes in a way that supports evolution and growth both individually and collectively.

I appreciate that Dr Pooja Sabharwal has dared to touch the subject which is otherwise untouched and succeeded to incorporate rich knowledge of traditional Indian medicine that is Ayurveda in purview of epigenetics through this manuscript. I am sure that this book will serve for new interventions with the eternal principals of Ayurveda which are appropriately placed in purview of epigenetics.

The author has explained the concepts of Ayurveda in the contest of epigenetics in a brilliant was based on her various presentations and publications on national as well as international platforms.

Let this book be an asset to the research fraternity around the globe for future collaborative studies in the filed of epigenetics and Ayurveda and let a new feather be added to Ayurveda research wing to make it stronger more for sharing its concepts with confidence.

I wish this book and author every success which she admirably deserves.

Prof. (Dr.) Vidula Gujjarwar

Director– Principal

FOREWORD

It gives me immense pleasure to write the foreword for this unique book entitled " Epigenetics and Ayurveda ". There is encouraging demand of contemporary understanding of fundamental concepts of Traditional Indian Medicine worldwide. "Genetics is an important part of the human story," "But epigenetics that is the other half of the equation." Epigenetics, which means "on top of genes," describes how the environment interacts with the genome to produce heritable changes resulting in phenotypic variation without altering the DNA of the genome. Epigenetics is recent and developing science. Many factors are causing epigenetical changes without change in DNA sequence. Epigenetics has many and varied potential medical applications as it tends to be multidimensional in nature. Modern science is realizing that epigenetic factors (i.e. diet, lifestyle, season, time of life, and individual tendencies) are directly influencing drug response. By taking the knowledge of modern science and combining it with the roots of Ayurveda, there is an opportunity to change the course of some of the most plaguing disorders of the modern world today.

I appreciate and congratulate Dr Pooja Sabharwal for her efforts of creating this manuscript for better understanding of Ayurvedic principals in purview of epigenetics which will certainly open doors for future collaborations among scientists & Ayurveda researchers. It is my proud privilege for being the part of various collaborative observational studies & publications with the author.

I believe that this book will be a milestone in understanding the fundamental concepts of Ayurveda among researchers in the field of genetics and epigenetics.

Dr. Rima Dada
MD, PhD, (Genetics), FNAMS, FIMSA, FASR Professor
Lab for Molecular Reproduction and Genetics
Department of Anatomy
AIIMS, New Delhi

●

Foreword

The science and art of medicine, which were initially one, having been separated in recent centuries, are now approaching reunification. In Ayurvedic literature, the living body is considered as amalgam of earth, water, fire, air and space and they comprisenot just the physical composition but also the mind and the spirit. That is, the individualas a whole includes structured matter, behavior, mind, soul, and consciousness, where the environment also providesa major contribution in the making of a person. Although classical anatomy viewed the human body is made up of systems, tissues and cells from gross to subtle level, medicine is now evolving to embrace the mind-body concept, which moves modern medicine along the path toward the age-old Ayurvedic concept.

Epigenetics is a new field of biology that is exploring the effect of the environment on heritable changes in the control of the expression of our genes, and thereby behavior of ourcells, and our daily health and mind-body functioning. The "environment" includes one's physical, social, and electromagnetic environment as well as daily and even one-time experiences, emotions, beliefs, perceptions, lifestyle, habits, behaviors, and mind-body practices such as meditation.

With the science of epigenetics we can begin to map out genes whose normal expression keeps us in a healthy state and we can begin to modulate the expression of other "bad" genes whose often-aberrant expression has plagued humans over the course of time.

In this book, Dr. Pooja Sabharwal brings out in much richer detail and depth her ideas regarding Ayurveda and epigenetics, which she has presented at international conferences during the past few years. She has done a commendable job of bridging between the advanced science of epigenetics, and the authoritatively wholistic science of Ayurveda, making connections for the first time between the ancient, time-tested practices of Ayurveda in the light of epigenetics. As a biomedical researcher with decades of interest in Ayurveda, I am inspired by her analysis, which brought to my awareness an abundance of opportunities for research uncovering epigenetic underpinnings of Ayurvedic practices, thereby integrating these two strands of medical science. I look forward to ongoing dialogue with Dr. Pooja Sabharwal leading to collaborative studies in this area. A beautiful unification of ancient and contemporary medical science is definitely happening as humanity's collective consciousness rises.

Sincerely,

John Fagan, Ph.D.
Professor of Molecular Biology
Maharishi University of Management
Chief Scientist and CEO
Health Research Institute
Fairfield, Iowa, USA

●

Foreword

It gives me immense pleasure to write the foreword for the manuscript "Epigenetics and Ayurveda". The phenotype of an individual is the result of complexgene–environment interactions in the current, past and ancestral environment, leading to lifelong remodeling of our epigenomes. Much attention is currently focusing on modulating hyper/hypo methylation of key in ammatory genes by dietary factors as an effective approach to cure or protect against cancer-in ammation. **Genes are absolutely not our fate**. They provide us useful information about the increased risk of a disease, but in most cases they will not determine the actual cause of the disease, or the actual incidence of somebody getting it. Phenotypic results will come from the complex interaction between the proteins and cells working with environmental factors, not driven directly by the genetic code".

Ayurveda is the study of life science. Ayu – meaning life and Veda – meaning science or knowledge. This science has been witnessed and practiced for 5000 years since the ancient Vedas were written. Ayurveda believes that the origin of disease is rooted in one key phrase, "Forgetting our true nature as spirit." I appreciate and congratulate Dr. Pooja Sabharwal for her efforts of creating this manuscript for explaining the Ayurvedic principals in purview of epigenetics in contemporary language. Scientists all around the globe are looking for multidisciplinary collaborative researches in the field of epigenetics. This manuscript will certainly serve as a eye opener for the scientific world.

(Dr. Ashok Sharma)

Faculty In–Charge
Division of Neueobio
Chemistry, AIIMS, New Delhi

Ayurveda has emerged as soft power of India around the globe. The fundamental concepts written in classical texts of Ayurveda has the potential to solve some of the world's most pressing health problems. This is the reason that Ayurveda is in demand not as complementary and alternative medicine but as mainstream medicine around the globe.

Need is to explore the soft power of Ayurveda. Research of fundamental concepts is real soft power of Ayurveda. Multidisciplinary collaborations to create evidence by doing rigorous research will open door to many scientific quests.

While doing research on fundamental concepts of Ayurveda in the field of oncology learned about epigenetics. After extensive understanding of epigenetics & its relation with Ayurveda the thought for writing this book was generated. The purpose of writing this book is to disseminate the knowledge of relative understanding of epigenetics and Ayurveda. Although research in form of observational studies to create evidence in this aspect is going on and various such kind of studies will be done to create maximum evidences.

Epigenetics the new science is evaluating the effect of the environment on cellular behavior. The "environment" includes every aspect i.e physical, social, and electromagnetic environment as well as beliefs, perceptions, lifestyle, habits, behaviors, and mind-body practices such as Pranic healing. Epigenetics is a new science while Ayurveda has been around 5000 years. According to both similar conclusions are their about impact of diet & environment on human body .

Modern science is realizing that epigenetic factors are directly linked with drug response. Integrating both the sciences and expanding the knowledge of science of epigenetics will help to eradicate various dreadful diseases. I feel gratitude towards my friends, collogues and family for supporting me while creating this manuscript.

This book covers various aspects of epigenetics science and its correlation with Ayurveda e.g Ayurvedic embryology in purview of epigenetics, Ayurinformatics and epigenetics, Ayurveda as bioenergetic medicine in purview of epigenetics. I look forward to receive opinions & suggestions from Ayurvedic and modern researchers for future collaborations in the field of epigenetics & Ayurveda.

New Delhi

11-06-2019

Dr. Pooja Sabharwal

(BAMS, MD, PHD, PGDHM, PGDYOGA, PGDAST, CFN)

●

CONTENTS

•

1   **W**hat is Epigenetics

Epigenetics is a recent branch of biology that is searching & exploring the effect of the environment & lifestyle on cellular behavior through changes the genetic expression. The "environment" consists of physical, social, and subtle environment as well as beliefs, perceptions, lifestyle, habits, behaviors, and mind-body practices such as Pranic healing. Epigenetics science has revealed that we can map out genes that keep us in a healthy state and remove those bad genes that have been killing humans over the course of time. There is real possibility to prevent and cure for many diseases including certain cancers & other dreadful diseases with the implementation of this science. It is the study of how we can change the expression of our genes without changing the sequence of the actual DNA or the genetic code.

There is a possibility to change the expression of our genes according to this new science. To elaborate the word epigenetics, "Epi" comes from the Greek word meaning *over*, *above*, or *outer*. According to this science there is possibility to change the genetics even without touching the genes. Two primary and interconnected epigenetic mechanisms - DNA methylation and covalent modification of histones are involved which are responsible for changes in genetic expression.

Epigenetic factor affects genes actually without changing the nucleotide sequence and which can be inherited through cell division. Epigenetic mechanisms involve the addition or removal of small chemical groups to or from DNA bases or chromatin.

Epigenetics is the science which reveals that we can even read the genetic code in different ways. With the help of which we can ultimately alter the path of disease cells, which begin as normal cells, to return to their proper behavior. This area of research is of that importance that the **National Institutes of Health has designated it as a major "Roadmap"** initiative to speed its development. This new science of epigenetics has the ability to explain the mechanisms that lead to many dreadful diseases like cancer, aging, heart disease, mental health and other conditions.

One of the scientist Omar Abdel-Wahab has explained this science as a growing field based on the study of genetic changes that are not part of the DNA code, and how these changes are responsible for dreadful diseases. It was believed till date that genetic inheritance is responsible for passing of genes from parents to child, but in fact, each time a cell in the body divides, genetic traits are passed on from that cell generation to the next. This concept is very well mentioned in classical text of Ayurveda which is explained in further chapters. Scientists are trying to learn the mechanisms involved in epigenetics.

In recent time scientists and researchers are very keenly indulged in exploring the two processes involved in epigenetics. In simple terms, epigenetics is the information that is passed down from parent cell to daughter cell but is not encoded in the DNA sequence. This field has become a important branch for research in many diseases like cancer.

Mechanisms explained in epigenetics are a normal part of many biological processes — for example, they allow stem cells to differentiate into more-specialized cell types but they also can lead to cancer and other diseases. A medical oncologist Omar Abdel-Wahab on the Leukemia Service and an investigator in the Human Oncology and Pathogenesis Program, is one of several Memorial Sloan Kettering researchers who is studying epigenetics specifically as it relates to cancer. He has mentioned that we are "just at the tip of the iceberg," but that research has already led to a handful of cancer drugs that work by targeting epigenetic changes.

There are two interconnected mechanisms involved in epigenetics that are methylation of DNA and modification of histones, proteins that bind to DNA. The impact of these two different mechanism is almost same. Which genes are expressed, or translated into proteins is impacted by these changes. These changes can silence genes by preventing DNA from being translated or activate genes that usually aren't turned on. According to the science of epigenetics DNA methylation occurs when a methyl group (a carbon atom with three hydrogen atoms attached) is added to a DNA strand. These mechanisms can influence the activity of gene at the transcriptional and post-transcriptional levels and/or at the translation level and post-translational modifications.

These epigenetic mechanisms with a potential of vast spectrum of consequences could result in more varieties of cell differentiations, morphogenesis, variability, and adaptability of an organism, which can be affected by both genetic and environmental factors. This science of epigenetics explains about the modifications of DNA, DNA-binding proteins, and histones, which are important in making changes in chromatin structure without changing in the nucleotide sequence of a given DNA. Few of these alterations could be transferred between generations. Such kind of modifications often happen during an organism's lifetime; however, these changes can be transferred to the next generation if they occur in germ cells.

Integrative medicine is a branch of science which prevents and maintain health by understanding the person's unique set of circumstances and addressing all aspects of physical, psychological, social, environmental, and spiritual influence. These treatment modalities were derived from traditional approaches that viewed the body as a single unit. Many research studies have indicated that thought and mental states are capable of affecting gene expression in various ways.

Scientists are trying to know the exact processes by which mind, thought, and consciousness arise within the brain have yet to be defined. In a recent study demonstrated how a synthetic mind-controlled transgene expression device enabled human brain activities and mental states (captured by an EEG headset) to regulate wireless optogenetic implants that radiated infrared frequency and ultimately programmed transgene expression in human designer cells implanted both in mice and in a semipermeable cultivation chamber.

In other studies, it has been shown that the autonomic nervous system (ANS), which is generally regarded as a system that cannot be voluntarily influenced, can in fact be brought under some conscious level of control. DNA methylation and histone modification which are main two epigenetic alterations can be regulated by external environmental factors in addition to the inherited genetic profile of an individual. These changes are deterministic of disease onset from childhood through adulthood.

The epigenome (i.e., the specific pattern of epigenetic mark including DNA methylation and histone modifications throughout the genome) causes the changes in physiological processes and psychological states inherent within everyone. Integrative Medicine has the potential to work at different levels, psychologically, physiologically, and/or directly at the level of the epigenome in the nucleus of a cell. The science of epigenetics is the future roadmap for integrative medicine.

References

- https://timesofindia.indiatimes.com/life-style/health-fitness/health-news/epigenetic-potential-of-nonpharmacological-intervention-in-oncology-an-integrated-approach/articleshow/71184650.cms.
- https://www.researchgate.net/publication/51737457_Genetics_epigenetics_and_pregenetics.
- https://1library.net/document/yr27jevz-cancer-and-epigenetics-interrelationship-in-prevention-and-cure.html
- https://www.sloankettering.edu/news/what-epigenetics.
- https://www.ncbi.nlm.nih.gov/pmc/articles/PMC5075137/
- https://www.researchgate.net/publication/304910902_Role_of_Epigenetics_in_Biology_and_Human_Diseases.
- https://unugp.education/dept-of-alternative-medicines/
- https://www.mskcc.org/news/what-epigenetics.
- https://www.ncbi.nlm.nih.gov/pmc/articles/PMC5339524/

2 Epigenetics and Ayurveda

Ayurveda science believes that "what you see, you become." It is the Ayurvedic understanding of epigenetics. The genetic expression can be influenced by the environment then it is good to have a healthy environment which is full in peace, love and joy and devoid of stress, violence and exhaustion. Ayurveda is science of life. The word Ayurveda is made up of two words, Ayu- meaning life and Veda- meaning science or knowledge. This traditional system of medicine has been witnessed and practiced for 5000 years since the ancient Vedas were written. The origin of disease according to Ayurveda is rooted in one key phrase, "Forgetting our true nature as spirit."

According to Sankhya philosophy, person desires to know its own nature merges with Prakriti. Which reveals the creation of the one's own soul. As per Ayurvedic perspective disease unfold when a person forgets their true nature as spirit. This happens at every incarnation. There is a store house of karma that is stored in the causal body at every incarnation When incarnation occurs the ahamkara takes form into an astral body where disturbance will take its origin.

The disturbances which occur at psychological level are known as vrittis in Ayurveda they upset the balance of a person which then manifests into the physical body as disease. In Charaka Samhita it is written, "The soul is essentially devoid of all pathogenecity" once we forget our true nature as spirit we then can start manifesting disease in the astral body. The concept of epigenetics is clearly visible in the ancient Ayurveda texts- Prakriti, Beej, Beejbhaga, Beejavyava, Sehej vyadhi/Adibala pravritta vyadhi, Shadgarbhakara bhava to name a few.

The Shadgarbhakara bhava are mentioned by Acharya Charak, Acharya Sushruta and Acharya Kashyap as- Matrija, Pitrija, Rasaja, Satmayaja, Atmaja and Sattvaja. Each factor when combined together results not only in organogenesis but also the psychological built of the progeny. With the very first glance at the somatic factors expressed by mother and father leads to development of soft organs and hard structures respectively. The rest forms the psyche. Ayurveda firmly puts its principles forward by being extremely specific for the progeny or race i.e. to be carried forward must be healthy. For females and developing fetus ancient texts are having abundant concepts- Ritukala Paricharya, Garbhadhana Ayu, Garbhadhana vidhi, Garbha Mamsanumasika Vridhhi, Douhrida, Mamsanumasika garbhini paricharya, Garbhopghatkara bhava, Garbha poshan etc. Whereas, especially for the offspring various Garbha samskara have been mentioned. But if these are not followed as described may lead to diseases enumerated in classics. Acharya Sushrut in Sutrasthana enlisted seven types of diseases- Adibala pravritta, Janmabala pravritta, Doshabala pravritta, Samghatabala pravritta, kalabala pravritta, Daivabala pravritta and Swabhavabala pravritta.

The disturbances that begin in the mind then start affect the physical body creating imbalance to the biological humors. There is certainly impact of maternal diet and lifestyle (Matura Ahara Vihara), and the age of the parents (Kala Ethnicity (Jati), familial characteristics (Satmya), as well as place of origin of an individual (Desha) to influence the transgenertional epigenetic inheritance.

Vitiation of Dosha because of defect in Gabhotpattikar bhava (ritu, kshetra, beej and ambu) leads to the impairment of the shape, colour, sensory as well as motor organs of the offspring. In Sushruta samhita, Sutrasthana, the seven types of diseases as Trividha dukha are mentioned. Among these Adibala pravritta vyadhi are the diseases which are congenital in origin and genetically determined like Dusta arsha, Prameha etc., are manifested due to vitiation of Shukra and Sonita of father and mother respectively.

The Acharya well states that it is the Beej that causes the congenital or hereditary disorders. Therefore, to prevent this Shodhana followed by Rasayana sevana is indicated so as to produce the healthiest possible offspring. During gametogenesis there is crossing over of genes between the chromosomes i.e. mutation and also the human body is constantly in interaction with the environment that can lead to some phenotypic changes which one some level may be beneficial by helping in adaptation; but may also be responsible for causing various congenital or hereditary disorders. the neurochemicals released due to negative emotions strain and damage the organs, whereas positive emotions release health-promoting chemicals.

Epigenetic changes are due to all molecular pathways modulating the expression of a genotype into a particular phenotype. In the recent past with the rapid growth of genetics, the meaning of the word has gradually narrowed. In present scientific world epigenetics has been defined accepted as "the study of changes in gene function that are mitotically and/or meiotically heritable and that do not actually touch the genetic code.

Current science is realizing that epigenetic factors (i.e. diet, lifestyle, season, time of life, and individual tendencies) are directly influencing drug response. Collaborating the current knowledge of contemporary science and combining it with the roots of Ayurveda, there are certainly good chances to change the course of some of the most dreadful disorders of the modern world today.

These modifications mainly include changes in diet, lifestyle, visual input, sensory stimulation, emotions, as well as many other environmental factors. Ayurveda science has explained taht any state that is not at Prakruti is a state of dis-ease and in order to treat this state there is need to know the psychological state of the patient, the nature of the disease and the nature of the modality available.

Any abnormality in human body is termed as disease which is made up of two words Dis means having a negative or reversing force. Ease means free from difficulty, effort, or trouble. So the term Dis-ease, is a negative reversal of the flow of ease. The traditional Indian medicine's holistic approach for treating the mind, body and soul as a complete person has the potential to solve some of the world's most pressing health problems. The contemporary science has seen this need for personalized medicine and Ayurveda offers the path which plays a key role towards disease prevention through diet and lifestyle.

Ayurveda science work at root cause by curing the fundamental causative factor of the disease instead of treating only symptom. The body will then be able to rid itself of the disease. The Charaka Samhita states, "The unwholesome combination of the sense organs with their objects, intellectual disturbaces (prajnaparadha) and transformation (parinama)– these are the main cause of diseases.

References

- http://www.ozarkresearch.org/site/epigenetics.html.

- *Epigenetics – What Ayurveda Already Knows By Gwen Diaz.* www. ayurveda college.com.

- Aguilera, O., Fernández, A. F., MuÛoz, A., & Fraga, M. F. 2010. Epigenetics and environment: A complex relationship. Journal of Applied [Manoj Jagtap et al: Enlightening Epigenetics Through Ayurveda And its Role In Future] 294 www.ijaar.in VOL II ISSUE III SEP-OCT 2015 Physiology, 109, 243-251. Retrieved July 24, 2012, fromhttp://jap.physiology.org/content/109/ 1/243.full.pdf (PDF - 582 KB).

- Bird, Adrian Perceptions of epigenetics Nature, Volume 447, Issue 7143, pp. 396-398 (2007).

- Gottlieb G "Epigenetic systems view of human development". Developmental Psychology 27 (1): 33–34.

- Maher B. Personal genomes: the case of the missing heritability. Nature 2008; 456:18–21.

- O'Connor, Anahad (11 March 2008). "The Claim: Identical Twins Have Identical DNA" New York Times. Retrieved 2 May 2010.

- Priya vrat Sharma Sushrut Samhita shaarirsthan 2/33 chaukhambha Visvabharati pg.134.

- Priya vrat Sharma Sushrut Samhita sharirsthana 5/3 chaukhambha Visvabharati pg.170.

- Prof. K.R. Srikantha Murty Astang Sangraha of Vagbhata 2/36 Chaukhambha Orientalia pg. 29.

- Sharma Anantram, editor. Sushrut Samhita Hindi Commentary. First edition. Varanasi: Chaukhamba Surbharti Prakashan, 2010; 2: 35,38. Sharma RK, Das B.

Charak Samhita, 2012; 1. Varanasi, U.P.: Chaukhamba Sanskrit Series Office, 2012; 391,398,399,400. Tripathi B. Ashtang Hridaya. 2012th ed. Delhi, Delhi: Chaukhamba Sanskrit Pratishthan, 2012; 344,348,349.

- Sharma RK, Das B. Charak Samhita. 2012 ed. Varanasi, U.P.: Chaukhamba Sanskrit Series Office, 2012; 2: 395, 396, 397.

- Sharma Anantram, editor. Sushruta Samhita Hindi Commentary. First edition. Varanasi: Chaukhamba Surbharti Prakashan, 2010; 2: 43.

- Sharma RK, Das B. Charak Samhita, 2012 ed. Varanasi, U.P.: Chaukhamba Sanskrit Series Office, 2012; 2: 370.

●

3 Epigenetics and Ayurvedic Embryology

While visiting a Ayurveda expert, the couples seeking to conceive are generally offered with unique suggestions. Till date most of the people understands the language of genetics, but according to science of epigenetics there is impact of experience, diet, and environment on genetic expression. The science of epigenetics explains the mechanisms of molecular changes including DNA methylation & histone modifications. The genes turned "on" and turned "off" when one is exposed to certain chemicals, psychological changes, environmental changes & diet can make one more or less susceptible to particular health problems.

"Genetics is only study of genetic code, an important aspect of human evolution while epigenetics, that is the study of expression of genes is equally important to know. Ayurveda which is traditional Indian system of medicine is based on *Triguna, Tanmatra, Tridosha, Saptdhatu, Oja, Agni, Ama* and *Srotas. Srotas* are the inner transport system of the body which provide platform to carry out the structural, functional and psychological activities of other important bio factors like metabolism, *Oja, Agni, Dhatu* etc.

Six procreative factors (*Shadgarbhkarabhavas*) play a prime role in formation of embryo (*Garbha*) and organogenesis. It is very clear that maternal and paternal factors are mostly responsible for anatomical development, while other factors like *Atma, Satva* are responsible for psychological development. The conglomeration of these procreative factors is must for healthy offspring. Any disturbance in the *Srotas* at the minute level (*Garbhaj Srotas*) *and* negligence towards six procreative factors either structurally, functionally and psychologically leads to the FOAD (foetal origin of adult diseases).

The concept of Shadgarbhakarabhavas explained by Ayurveda seers and the concept of FOAD (foetal origin of adult diseases) has been attaining considerable importance these days. The unfavourable conditions during life in the womb and in childhood along with affecting health in childhood, also predispose to increased risk of diseases in adulthood. The Ayurveda scholars has mentioned some unique preprations for the healthy progeny and safe delivery which includes proper preparation of parents, Punsavana-samskara, Masanumasik Paricharya, avoidance of Garbhaupghatkarabhava, proper use of Kumaragara Sutikagara, Dhupana, Raksha karma, Seemantonayana, Jatkarma-samskara etc.

Incorporation of these principles in daily routine practice, natural delivery can be ensured which is free from various complications & accompanied with good maternal health, a healthy progeny with good immunity and ultimately good lactation which will help in proper growth of the baby.

Ayurveda which is holistic health science, not only deal with preventive and curative aspects of health but also has recommendations for healthy progeny. Shadgarbhakara-bhav (Six procreative factors of progeny) have been propounded in the Ayurvedic classics viz. Matrija (mother), Pitrija (father), Atmaja (soul), Satmyaja (wholesome practices by mother), Rasaja (diet of the mother) and Satvaja (psychological health of the parents).

Healthy mother, father, proper diet of the mother, practice of wholesome living and dietary regimen and healthy mind, psychological status of parents & good deeds of soul in previous incarnation play a important role in achieving healthy offspring, that is how a disease free nation can be structured. Six procreative factors (Shadgarbhkarabhavas) are play a prime role in formation of embryo (Garbha) and organogenesis.

These shadbhavas are not only responsible for the structural growth of foetus but they play also important role in the development of psychological, spiritual and emotional factors. It is very clear that maternal and paternal factors are mostly responsible for anatomical development, while other factors like Atma, Satva are responsible for psychological development. The conglomeration of these procreative factors is must for healthy offspring. Any disturbance in the Srotas at the minute level (Garbhaj Srotas) and negligence towards six procreative factors either structurally, functionally and psychologically leads to the FOAD (foetal origin of adult diseases).

Concept of FOAD (Foetal Origins of Adult Disease):

David Barker's theory has been popularized as the "Barker hypothesis," or "Foetal Origins of Adult Disease" (FOAD). This theory is based on the fact of "developmental plasticity" which means that a single genotype is influenced by specific intrauterine events, has the capability to produce different phenotypes.

Various studies data reveals that 3 – 5% of all births result in congenital malformations, 20 – 30% of all infant deaths are due to genetic disorders, and almost 50 percent of post-neonatal deaths are due to congenital malformations, most of pediatric hospital admissions are for children with genetic disorders, most of children with other congenital malformations, rest adult hospital admissions are for genetic causes, and also mental retardation has a genetic basis.

A good percentage of all chronic diseases (heart, diabetes, arthritis), which occur in the adult population are due to defect in genetic component. The **foetal origin of adult diseases hypothesis** (differentiated from the developmental origins of health and disease hypothesis, which highlighed environmental conditions both before and immediately after birth) explained the concept that the period of gestation has significant impacts on the developmental health and wellbeing outcomes for an individual ranging from infancy to adulthood.

Three characteristics latency, persistency & programming mainly have impact on the effect of foetal origin . **Latency**, wherein effects may not be apparent until much later in life; **persistency**, whereby conditions resulting from a foetal effect continue to exist for a given individual; and **genetic programming**, which explains the 'switching on' or 'off' of a specific gene due to prenatal environment. This epidemiologist published his findings proposing a direct link between prenatal nutrition and late-onset coronary heart disease. His observations revealed that the poorest areas of England were the same areas with the highest rates of heart disease, unveiling the predictive relationship between low birth weight and adult disease.

Since Barker's initial findings, the results have been replicated in diverse populations of Europe, Asia, North American, Africa, and Australia. The FOAD hypothesis mentioned that events during early development have a sound impact on one's risk for development of future adult disease. Factors like low birth weight, a surrogate marker of poor fetal growth and nutrition, is linked to many diseases like coronary artery disease, hypertension, obesity, and insulin resistance.

In recent past studies it has been seen that theses observations by david barker stands true.

FOAD concept understanding is really very important for health care professionals and policy makers as it will make this issue a high healthcare priority and implement preventative measures and treatment for those at higher risk for chronic diseases. David Barker's keen observations have been popularized as the "Barker hypothesis," or "Fetal Origins of Adult Disease" (FOAD). For the first time it was noted that low birth weight (LBW) serves as proxy not just for fetal, but also adult health.

As revealed by many studies LBW is associated with a host of chronic diseases ranging from coronary artery disease (CAD), Type II diabetes mellitus (T2DM), cancer, and osteoporosis to various psychiatric illnesses . The concept of FOAD is based on the premise of "developmental plasticity"—a single genotype, influenced by specific intrauterine events, has the capability to produce different phenotypes. Specific developmental periods during intrauterine life effects the foetal life which may manifest during adult life. The adversity faced by foetus due to malnutrition will cause remodeling thereby altering structure and function of various organs to preserve neurodevelopment and promote survival. Such changes prepare the fetus for extrauterine life where additional stressors may be encountered. This is the science behind epigenetics.

The FOAD theory proposed by David Barker was supported by large birth registries and human cohorts where gestating women and their offspring faced severe malnutrition in the form of famines. In these studies record of birth history of men & women were taken & later these subjects were identified in later life. This is how the investigator correlated birth weight and childhood growth and the later onset of diseases in adulthood.

Numerous epidemiological studies across various cultures and ethnicities support the link between LBW and future adult disease. Those with "normal" birth weights, appropriate for gestational age (AGA), may still be at risk which depends on the type, timing, and duration of the original infection. Any sort of alterations in diet composition, inflammation, infection, glucocorticoids, hypoxia, stress, and toxins also play a vital role in shaping the adult phenotype. The studies found tends to focus on the LBW, or small for gestational age (SGA) baby, special consideration must be given to the stressed AGA, large for gestational age (LGA), and premature neonate. The transgenerational and socio-economic implications of FOAD have far-reaching repercussions that cannot be underestimated; as further research is still needed to know in depth about its complexities. *Ayurveda* seers have elaborated the importance of the concept of FOAD (foetal origin of adult diseases) has been attaining much attention as these factors not only do unfavourable conditions during life in the womb and in childhood affect health in childhood, they also predispose to increased risk of diseases in adulthood.

Epigenetics & FOAD (Foetal origins of Adult Disease):

Epigenetics is the study of changes in the organisms which is caused by modification of gene expression. With this branch of science, it can be described anything other than DNA that is influencing the development of an organism. Genotype and Phenotype are two important and basic aspects in this context.

The genotype is the genetic make up of an individual

whereas Phenotype is the set of observable characters of the individual resulting from the interaction of its genotype. The concept of foetal origins of adult diseases describes *in utero* programming, or adaptation to a range of adverse environmental conditions that ultimately leads to increased susceptibility to age-related diseases later in life. The exact mechanism of this biological memory is still unclear, but science of epigenetics is revealing evidences for the same. The increased incidences of chronic diseases and involvement of multiple organ systems that is observed is analogous to the decline in resistance to disease that is typical of normal aging. The overall environment over the course of a lifetime can induce increasing epigenetic dysregulation. **Epigenetics**, which means "**upon the top of genes**," explains how the environment interacts with the genome to produce heritable changes resulting in phenotypic variation without touching the DNA of the genome.

"Pregnancy should be by choice not by chance". Counseling prior to conception can play a vital role not only in achieving the goal of a healthy progeny, but also in preventing congenital and genetic disorders. *Garbhakarabhavas* are carriers of the organogenesis and other traits to the foetus. These traits are similar to the traits carried by chromosomes/ genes as per contemporary concepts, embryogenesis, foetal growth, and development. The requirement for healthy progeny includes proper preparation of parents, *Punsvanasamskara, Masanumasikparicharya,* avoidance of *Garbhaupghatkarabhav,* proper use of *Kumaragara, Sutikagara, Dhupana, Raksha Karma, Seemantonayana, Jatakarmasamskara* etc.

Impact of *Shadgarbhakarabhavas* (six procreative factors) in genesis of *Garbha* (foetus):

"Shukrashosheetjeevsanyogetukhalukukshigate Garbha-iteeabhidheeyate."

Shukra & *shonita* unite in the womb of the mother than it is called as *Garbha* or Embryo.

"Shukrashosheet Garbhashayasthaatamaprakrutvika-rasamudayatmasamayogavahi Garbhaitichutye".

Samayoga means proper union of *shuksra, shonit, mana, atma & Panchma-habhoots*. This includes union of sixteen *vikaras* and eight *prakruti* also. This union has happened according to *ati-indriyatwatvat, ati-sukshmatvat*, all minute structures mix with each other.

As per the *Ayurvedic* concepts of *Shareer* (Embryo-genesis), each procreative factor contributed in the physical and mental growth and development of certain structures as well as functions of the body, which are tabulated in Table 1. Perfection of all these procreative factors in turn of their assigned structures and functions leads to a healthy progeny [Table 1].

The *Matrija, Pitriju,* and *Atmaja* Bhavas cannot be changed as they come from the parents and *Poorvajanma Samskaras* (as a result of the code of conduct), respectively, but the other three Bhavas-factors, namely, *Satmyaja, Rasaja* and *Sattvaja Bhavas*, practiced properly can actually modify the intrauterine environment and psychosomatic health of the mother, which produce a great impact on the foetus. These days it is a known fact now that environmental factors can influence the genome.

According to conventional medical science, there are three phases of intrauterine growth. Zygote, embryo, and foetus. Genetic constitution of the foetus, nutritional status of the mother, placental status, uterine capacity, exposure to infections, and toxic factors (i.e., rubella, alcohol, narcotics) affect the intrauterine growth of the foetus.

The first, that is, the zygote phase—Period-I (weeks 1–2 after fertilization) consists of cell division and implantation of this cell mass in the uterus. During the second, that is, the embryonic phase or Period II (weeks 3–8) most of the organ systems develop and in the third, that is, foetal phase/ PeriodIII (weeks 9–38) further growth and elaboration of the organ systems takes place. *Shadgarbhakarabhavas* (Six procreative factors) are play a prime role in formation of *Garbha* (embryo) and organogenesis. It is very clear that maternal and paternal factors are mostly responsible for anatomical development, while other factors like *Atma, Satva* are responsible for psychological development. The conglomeration of these procreative factors is must for healthy offspring. Any disturbance in the *Srotas* at the minute level (*Garbhaj Srotas*) *and negligence towards six procreative factors* either structurally, functionally and psychologically leads to the FOAD (foetal origin of adult diseases).

Table 1.

Pro-creative factors	Features developed from six procreative factors
Matrijabhav (Maternal)	*twaka, rakta, mansa, meda, nabhi, hridaya, klom, yakrita, pleeha, vrikka, basti, pureeshadhan, aamashaya, pakwashaya, uttaguda, adharguda, Kshudrantra, sthulantra, vapa, vapavahan*[22], **Majja,** Garbhashaya[23], **Krishna mandal**[24], etc.
Pitrijabhav (Paternal)	*kesha,smashru, nakha, loma, danta, asthi, sira, snayu, dhamni, shukra*[25], **suklamandal** etc.

Atmaja (Soul)	Ayu, atmagyana, Mana, indriyan, prana, apana, preran, dharan, aakritivishesh, swaravishesh, varnavishesha, sukha, dukkha, ichchha, dwesh, chetna, dhriti, budhi, smriti, ahamkara, prayatna etc.
Satmyaja (Wholesome ness)	Aaroggya, analasya, aloluptwa, indriyaprasada, swara, sampat, varna sampat, beejasampat, prahasha etc.
Rasaja (Nutrition factor)	Sharirabhinirvritti, sharirabhivridhi, prananubandhi, tripti, pushti, utsaha etc.
Satvaja (Mind)	Bhakti, sheel, shaucha, dwesha, smriti, moha, tyaga, matsarya, shaurya, bhaya, krodha, tandra, utasaha, taikshana, mardava, gambhirya, anavasthitva etc[26].

Srotodusti of *Garbha*:

Srotas are the inner transport system of the body which provide platform to carry out the structural, functional and psychological activities of the human body like metabolism. There is no direct reference available in classical *Ayurvedic* literature about srotas in the aspect of *Garbha* (embryo).There are four types of *Srotodiushti* available in *Ayurvedic* text. These are *Atipravritta, Sanga, Siragranthi*and *Vimarg gaman*. Any disturbance in the *Srotas* at the minute level (*Garbha*) due to those four types of *Srotodushti* either structurally functionally, and psychologically may lead to FOAD.For example, if there is *Atipravritti*, it may lead to cancer.

Concept of Genetics in *Ayurveda*:

The word genetics derived from ancient Greek word "Genetikos" mean to genesis or origin. **Genetics** is the study of genes, genetic variation, and heredity in living organisms.

Science of genetics in *Ayurveda* may appear a new topic but ancient *Ayurvedic* scholars like *Charaka* and *Sushruta* understood very well the Principles of heredity and nature of traits or characters. They knew the fundamentals of Genetics i.e. the factors determining the sex of a child, genetic defect in a childlike lameness. *Acharya Charaka* has described the whole genetics in three genetic units in the form of *Beej* (Germinal cell), *Beejbhag* (Chromosome) and *Beejbha-gavyava* (Gene).

He has explained that due to *vikriti* of *bija*, *bijabhaga* and *bijabhagavayava* of the couple, there will be *vikriti* or *vyapada* in the child depending on gender. *Adibalapravritta*[1] diseases, groups of illnesses which are attributed defects inherent in either the *Shukra* (the male reproductive element) or *Shonita* (female reproductive element) which form the primary factors of being.

There are six factors which are taking part in the formation of embryo and various body parts. All the soft structures i.e. heart, spleen, intestine, rectum, muscles, blood, lipid, bone marrow, umbilicus etc. ofthe foetus are derived from the mother, called *Matrija bhava*. Likewise, all stable or hardparts i.e. hairs, vein, arteries, nails, bones,beard, sperm etc. Of foetus are derived from the father, called *Pitrija bhava*.

Just like above *Atmaja, Satmayaja, Satvaja & Rasajabhavas* are also taking part in the formationof a foetus in the uterus. *Ayurveda* Science had basic or fundamental knowledge on genetics since very early time period when there was no existence of concept like Chromosomes, genes, DNA, genome etc.

Our classical Scholars have explained the facts that genetic disorders are not due to any defect in the mother or, the father but in the ovum or sperm of the parents, therefore they advised some ritualistic therapy and cleansing (*Shodhana*) of the male and female body before planning to have a child and to take rejuvenation therapy to restore health which prevents the appearance of genetic disorder. Whatever our *Acharyas* have told in our classics about genetics should be scientifically validated to give better explanations worldwide.

Transgenerational Inheritance of Epigenetic Effect and Ayurveda

Many factors can cause epigenetic and developmental epigenetic changes - Exercise, diet, drugs alcohol chemicals in the living space or workplace, Medications. These environmental factors are only a few examples of things that can cause epigenetic changes.

Many other environmental factors, known and unknown can cause epigenetic changes. In 2008, the National Institutes of Health announced that $190 million had been utilized for epigenetics research over the next five years. Government officials noted that epigenetics has the potential to explain mechanisms of aging, human development, and the origins of cancer, heart disease, mental illness, as well as several other conditions.

Scientists, like Randy Jirtle, PhD, of Duke University Medical Center think epigenetics may ultimately turn out to have a greater role in disease than genetics. According to Ayurveda union of shukra (sperm) and shonita (ovum) into garbhashay (uterus) along with aatma (soul) is called as garbha (embryo). Other factors like ritu, kshetra, ambu and beeja are responsible for formation of garbha.

Any abnormality in these factors can cause congenital anomalies. Other factors like diet, exercise, alcohol, stress, exertion etc can effect both mother and fetus. Garbha is known to be formed by six factors like matruja, pitruja, rasaja, satvaja, saatmyaja and aatmaj. These are actually combination of genetic, psychological and nutritional factors. Many of these factors can cause congenital anomalies like vitiated beeja i.e. shukra and shonita causes fetal defects. Many of diseases like prameha, kushta are said to be caused by beeja dushti which later seen in adult life. Ayurveda has mentioned about garbha upghaatkar bhaav meaning factors causing abnormalities to fetus. These factors include exertion, trauma, journey, keeping awake at nights, suppression of urges, fasting, abnormal postures, hearing unpleasant sounds etc. Genetics is science of genes. Genes are parts of chromosomes situated in nucleus. Abnormality in genes and nchromosome causes many diseases and birth defects. Epigenetics is branch of science which deals with cellular and physiological traits that are heritable by daughter cells and not caused by changes in the DNA sequence.

Epigenetical changes are caused by some factors. For example In one study, Marcus Pembrey and colleagues observed that the paternal grandsons of Swedish men who were exposed during preadolescence to famine in the 19th century were less likely to die of cardiovascular disease. The fact that food was plentiful, then diabetes mortality in the grand children increased, suggesting that this was a trans-generational epigenetic inheritance. A more advanced study, where 114 monozygotic twins and 80 dizygotic twins were analyzed for the DNA methylation status of around 6000 unique genomic regions, came to the conclusion that epigenetic similarity at the time of blastocyst splitting may also contribute to phenotypic similarities in monozygotic co-twins.

Such kind of studies supports the fact that microenvironment at early stages of embryonic development can be quite important for the establishment of epigenetic marks for considerable changes even in adulthood. Genomic imprinting which is a phenomenon in mammals where the father and mother contribute different epigenetic patterns for specific genomic loci in their germ cells is associated with some human disorders. One of the case of imprinting in human disorders is that of Angelman syndrome and Prader-Willi syndrome, these both can be produced by the same genetic mutation, chromosome 15q partial deletion, and the particular syndrome that will develop depends on whether the mutation is inherited from the child's mother or from their father. This is due to the presence of genomic imprinting in the region.

Not only the maternal factor is responsible for epigenetic changes to offspring. Various experimental studies with rats have shown the crop fungicide vinclozolin can cause susceptibility to cancer and kidney defects, both of which can be transferred to offspring through methylation changes. Similarly, in another medical experiment, researchers discovered that cocaine-using mice passed memory problems on to three generations of descendants. It is becomimg much clearer that factors like Exercise, Diet, Nicotine, Alcohol, Chemicals in the living space or workplace & Medications can induce epigenetical changes which may land up into diseases which may be transgenerational. Many of factors are still unknown. Ayurveda has mentioned above factors as hetu i.e. etiological factors. Also Ayurveda mentions that exposure to these factors during pregnancy will cause congenital anomalies.

Epigenetics is new and developing science. Many factors are causing epigenetical changes without actually having change in DNA sequence. Epigenetics has many and different potential medical applications as it tends to be multidimensional in nature. Transgenerational diseases occur due to these epigenetical changes. Ayurveda science has stated many factors causing diseases and congenital birth defects. Many of the etiological factors mentioned in Ayurveda science now can be explained in the language of epigenetics.

References:

- https://www.theatlantic.com/politics/archive/2014/03/epigenetics-the-controversial-science-behind-racial-and-ethnic-health-disparities/430749/
- https://www.worldwidejournals.com/indian-journal-of-applied-research-(IJAR)/article/impact-of-six-procreative-factors-on-srotodusti-of-garbha-in-manifestation-of-foad-foetal-origin-of-adult-disease/MTY0NzY=/?is=1
- https://en.wikipedia.org/wiki/Fetal_origins_hypothesis
- https://www.ncbi.nlm.nih.gov/pmc/articles/PMC3215361/
- https://www.ncbi.nlm.nih.gov/pmc/articles/PMC4608552/
- Verma V https://www.ncbi.nlm.nih.gov/pmc/articles/PMC3215361/andana, Gehlot Sangeeta. Review on concept of srotas. Int. J. Res. Ayurveda Pharm. 2014; 5(2): 232-234 *http://dx.doi.org/10.7897/2277-4343.05246.*
- Gaikwad Rutuja, Healthy Progeny through Ayurveda, Journal of Dental & Medical Sciences (IORS-JDMS) e-ISSN:2279-0853, P-ISSN:2279-0861. Vol.13, Issue1 Ver. IX. (Feb.2014), pp.115-119.
- Darokar Shrikant Bhaurao: Concept of Shad Garbhakara Bhavas in Ayurveda. International Ayurvedic Medical

Journal {online} 2017 {cited September, 2017} http://www.iamj.in/posts/images/upload/735_741.pdf.

- Robinson A, Linden MG. Clinical Genetic Handbook. Boston: Blackwell Scientific Publications; 1993.
- Berry RJ, Buehler JW, Strauss LT, Hogue CJ, Smith JC. Birth weight-specific infant mortality due to congenital abnormalities, 1960 and 1980Public Health Rep 1987; 102:171-81.
- Hoekelman RA, Pless IB. Decline in mortality among young American during the 20th century: Prospects for reaching national mortality reduction goals for 1990. Paediatrics 1988; 82:582-95.
- Scriver CR, Neal JL, Saginur R, Clow A. The frequency of genetic disease and congenital malformation among patients in a paediatric hospital. Can Med Assoc J 1973; 108:1111-5.
- Emery AE, Rimoin DL. Principles and Practice of Medical Genetics. 2nd ed. New York: Churchill Livingstone; 1990.
- Schneider KA. Counselling about Cancer: Strategies for Genetic Counsellors. Dennis port, Massachusetts: Graphic Illusions; 1994.
- Weatherall DJ. The New Genetics and Clinical Practice. 2nd ed. Oxford: Oxford University Press; 1985.
- Weatherall DJ. Heart, diabetes arthritis which occur in the adult populations have a significant genetic component. The New Genetics and Clinical Practice. 2nd ed. Oxford: Oxford University Press; 1985.
- Advisory committee on the Biological Effects of Ionizing Radiation. The Effect on Populations of Exposure to Low Levels of Ionizing Radiation.
- Washington DC: NR Council, NAS, National Academy Press; 1980.
- Almond, Douglas; Currie, Janet (2011). "Killing Me

Softly: The Foetal Origins Hypothesis." The Journal of Economic Perspective. 25(3): 153-172. Doi:10.1257/jep. 25.3.153.

- Barker, David; Osmond, C. (1986). "Infant mortality, childhood nutrition, and ischaemic heart diseasein England and Wales". Lancet. **327**:1077–1081. *doi: 10.1016/s0140-6736(86)91340-1.*

- Paul, Annie Murphy (2011). Origins: how the nine months before birth shape the rest of our lives (1st Free Press trade pub. ed.). New York: Free Press. ISBN 978-0743296632.

- Shiksha Rana: Prerequisites of Ayurveda In Healthy Progeny. International Ayurvedic Medical Journal {online} 2017 {cited June, 2017} http://www.iamj.in/posts/images/upload/2137_2144. pdf.

- Agnivesha, Charaka Samhita, revised by charaka and Dradhabala, edited by Kashinath shastri, Gnagasahaya Pandey, Chaukhambha Sanskrit Sansthan, Varanasi, vol.1, reprint 2007, Sharirsthana 4/5, pg.757.

- Sushrut Samhita of maharsisushrut, Edited with Ayurved tattva Sandipika by Kaviraj Ambikadutta Shastri forword by pranajivana Manekechand Mehta. Chaukhambha Sunskritsansthan, Varanasi, reprint Edition 2005, vol.1, Sharirsthana 2/34, pg.-146.

- Agnivesha, Charaka Samhita, revised by Charaka and Dradhabala, edited by Priyavrit Sharma, Chaukhambha Orientalia, Varanasi, vol.1, reprint 2011, Sharirsthana 3/17, pg.-753.

- Dhimankamini, Kumar Abhimanayu, Dhiman K.S., Shad Garbhakara Bhavas Vis-Œ-vis Congenital and Genetic Disorders; AYU Journal; April 2010, DOI: 10.4103/0974-8520.72384. Source: Pub Med.

- Agnivesha, Charaka Samhita, revised by charaka and Dradhabala, edited by Priyavrit Sharma, Chaukhambha

Orientalia, Varanasi, vol.1, reprint 2011, Sharirsthana 3/6, pg.742.

- Astang Samgraha of Vridha Vagbhatta with the Sasilekha Sunskrit Commentary by Indu, edited by Shivprasad Sharma, Chowkhambha Sunskrit Series office, Varanasi, Vol.1, Sharirsthana 5/14, pg300.

- Astang Samgraha of Vridha Vagbhatta with the Sasilekha Sunskrit Commentary by Indu, edited by Shivprasad Sharma, Choukhambha Sunskrit Series office, Varanasi, Vol.1, Sharirsthana 5/49, pg.304.

- Kasyapa Samhita or Vridha Jivaka tantra by Vridha Jivaka revised by Pandit Hemraj Sharma Vidyotini Hindi Commentary, Chaukhambha Sanskrit Sansthan, Varanasi, Edition: Reprint, 2010, Sharirsthana, 3/4, pg.72.

- Agnivesha, Charaka Samhita, revised by charaka and Dradhabala, edited by Priyavrit Sharma, Chaukhambha Orientalia, Varanasi, vol.1, reprint 2011, Sharirsthana 3/10-13, pg.746-748.

- Gayathri H. & Byresh A: Sroto Vaigunya, Sroto Dushti And Sroto Viddha – A Conceptual Study. International Ayurvedic Medical Journal {online} 2017 {cited July, 2017}, http://www.iamj.in/posts/images/upload/2517_2524.pdf.

- www.enwikipedia.org/wiki/genetics assed on 03 July 2016, time 11.05 am.

- Griffiths, Anthony J. F.; Miller, Jeffrey H.; Suzuki, David T.; Lewontin, Richard C.; Gelbart, eds. (2000)." Genetics and the Organism: Introduction". *An Introduction to Genetic Analysis* (7th ed.). New York: W. H. Freeman. ISBN 0-7167-3520-2.

- Agnivesha, Charaka Samhita, revised by charaka and Dradhabala, edited by Kashinath shastri, Gnagasahaya Pandey, Chaukhambha Sanskrit sansthan, Varanasi, vol.1, reprint 2007, Sharirsthana 4/30, pg.877-878.

- Sushrut Samhita of maharsisushrut, Edited with Ayurved tattva Sandipika by Kaviraj Ambikadutta Shastri forword by pranajivana Manekechand Mehta. Chaukhambha Sunskritsansthan, Varanasi, reprint Edition 2005, vol.1, Sutra sthana 24/6, pg.100.
- Triwedi Priyanka: Genetics in Ayurveda: View of Ancient Scholars. International Ayurvedic medical Journal {online} 2016 {cited 2016 July} http://www.iamj.in/posts/images/upload/2623_2627.pdf.
- Kara Calkins, Sherin U. Devaskar; Curr Probl Pediatr Adolesc Health Care. 2011 Jul; 41(6): 158–176.doi: 10.1016/j.cppeds. 2011.01.001.
- Almond Douglas, Mazumdar Bhashkar."Health Capital and the Prenatal Environment: The Effect of Ramadan Observance During Pregnancy", American Economic Journal Applied Economics 3(4): 56-85. October 2011; DOI: 10.1257/app.3.4.56.
- Velasquez-Manoff, Moises. "Should You Bring Your Unborn Baby to Work?". *The Atlantic*. The Atlantic Magazine. Retrieved 12 November 2015.
- DNA signature in Ice Storm babies: Prenatal maternal stress exposure to natural disasters predicts epigenetic profile of offspring". *Science Daily.com*. Retrieved 13 November 2015.
- Harkiran Nehra: Ayurveda, Genetics and Genomics: An Integrative Approach to Traditional and Basic Sciences. International Ayurvedic Medical Journal {online} 2017 {cited March, 2017} mm .
- Reid F. Thompson, Francine H. Einstein, Epigenetic Basis for fetal Origins of Age-Related Disease, Journal of women's Health, Vol.19, No. 3, 25 March, 2010, http://doi.org/10.1089/jwh. 2009.1408.

4 | Intervention of Ayurveda in Oncology in Purview of Epigenetics

Cancer is the second most common dreadful cause of death and accounts for nearly 1 of every 4 deaths worldwide. As per the report of the World Health Organization worldwide, there were 14 million new cancer cases and 8.2 million cancer-related deaths in 2015.

Who has reported that the annual worldwide cancer cases will rise from 14 million in 2015 to 22 million by 2030, which is itself very scary situation. Actually diet & lifestyle has direct link with cancer prevention & care. Consumption of plant based diet, organic food, stress free life, meditation, exercise, low inflammatory status can prevent cancer growth. Cancer is manifested in mainly three stages initiation, promotion, and progression. The process of initiation involves a primary mutation in the DNA which leads to a cell with increased potential for growth but actually this is still dependent on additional genotypic and epigenetic changes due to faulty diet & lifestyle for achieving complete transformation to malignancy.

Due to lack of these co-required epigenetic changes, the mutation once happen at initial stage will not manifest into cancer. As the process of initiation is influenced by epigenetic changes. On the other hand, epigemone which is influenced by diet Alternatively, changes already induced within the epigenome due to certain factors may promote cellular transformation upon a subsequent DNA mutagenic event. So the epigenetic factor is involved with the genetic factor. The process of modifications that occur on histone N-terminal tails and on DNA are shown together with the enzymes that lay down and remove the marks. They turn oncogenic due to the process of deregulation.

Certain genotoxic carcinogenic agents start the process of initiation and they directly damage the DNA. The process of promotion further involves proliferation of previously intitated cells under the influence of epigenetic process.

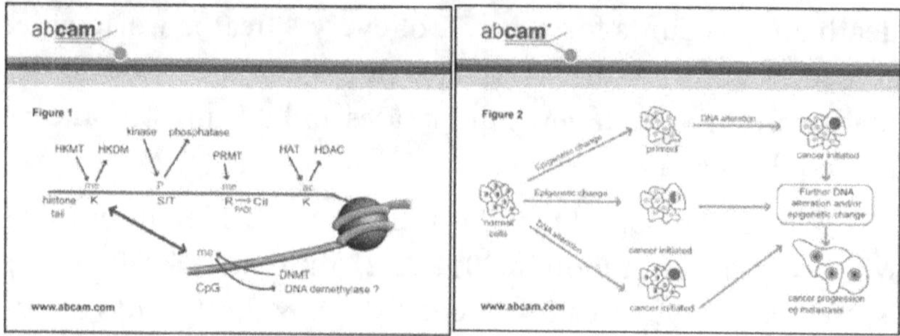

The modifications which occur on histone N-terminal tails and on DNA have been shown together with the enzymes that lay down and remove the marks. Any kind of deregulation of these enzymes has the potential to be oncogenic. Genetic & epigenetic changes are responsible for progression of the development of that early cancerous clone of cells into a fully malignant phenotype.

The classical literature of Ayurveda has described two related categories of swellings, one inflammatory (arbuda) and the other non-inflammatory (granthi), though this division is somewhat not definite. malignant form is considered as Arbuda. There is explanation in the ancient Ayurvedic medical texts that arbuda is due to secondary outcome of a chronic inflammatory pathology. Arbuda and granthi come under the category of diseases called "Üopha". Ýopha can be correlated as an "inflammatory swelling. Sushruta has described the arbuda as "The disturbed doshas established in any part of the body afflict the mamsa dhatu and produce a swelling which is fixed, hardened, only slightly painful, circular, broad-based, slowly growing and does not suppurate." That is how it is like that Üopha, especially when it persists in chronic form, predisposes the individual to develop arbuda. In Charaka's explanation on the treatment of vŒtarakta (gouty arthritis), a chronic inflammatory disease affecting the joints of the body, arbuda is described as sometimes occurring as a complication.

CANCER IN ADULT LIFE IN PURVIEW OF TRANSGENERATIONAL EPIGENETIC INHERITENCE

The science of genetics has even explained that maternal and paternal chromosomes are not responsible for the phenotype, but epigenetic factors influence these changes. A sequence of questions can be asked from the expectant mother for her dietary regimen as it will effect the unborn child. It is becoming more and more evident that not only her children, but her grandchildren and subsequent generations will be affected by her nutrition. What the mother eats may not only affect her descendants as they develop, but potentially affect them throughout their adult lives. The early intrauterine environment of a developing child can talk to its genome by epigenetic means. Environmental factors trigger changes to epigenetic tags on our genome, which causes the way genes are expressed. These changes on the genome can be transferred from cell to cell as we replace damaged body tissue. When such changes occur inside the egg or sperm cells, they can pass through to the next generation. Therefore, along with inheriting our genes, we also inherit their modes of expression. Epidemiologist David Barker proposed the theory of foetal origins of adult disease, later the theory was denoted as "Barker's hypothesis". In 1986, Barker published findings proposing a direct link between prenatal nutrition and late-onset of cancer. He also unveiled the predictive relationship between low birth weight and adult disease. In Ayurveda the concept of FOAD (foetal origin of adult diseases) has been attaining considerable attention as not only do unfavourable conditions during life in the womb and in childhood affect health in childhood, they also predispose to increased risk of diseases in adulthood.

In case of breast cancer there is strongest evidence for cancer and FOAD exists as per the scientific studies. One of the case-control study revealed that those individuals at birth who weighed less than 2.5 kg were half as likely as those who weighed greater than 4 kg to subsequently develop breast cancer. In a cohort of 2221 British women, a birth weight >3.5 kg was associated with an increased risk for cancer, specifically pre-menopausal breast cancer, even after adjusting for confounders.

It was stated by one scientist that in utero exposure to high levels of estrogens, either endogenous or exogenous, increased the number of stem cells and/or mitogenic activity of undifferentiated breast tissue. Based upon this theory it has been observed that mothers with advanced age, dizygotic gestations, or macrocosmic or preterm babies demonstrate higher concentrations of estrogen.

As a result, their fetuses were at an increased risk for breast cancer development. Similarly it has been seen that mothers diagnosed with pregnancy-induced hypertension have decreased estrogen concentrations, and therefore, their offspring are relatively protected from breast cancer. In another study it was noticed that pre-eclampsia/eclampsia was associated with a substantially lower breast cancer rate.

Interestingly in one of the study it was found that women who are taller in childhood and have higher growth rates seem to carry an even higher risk. It was observed that for every

5-cm increase in height, there is an 11% increase in breast cancer, thus highlighting growth factors, such as the insulin-like growth factor, potentially yet another carcinogenic factor. Cancer is a complex and dreadful disease. Only genetic mutations and environmental triggers are not sufficient to explain the pathogenesis and the rising incidence of cancer, obesity, T2DM & other complex diseases. Epigenetics, which means "beyond the genetics" explains how the diet, lifestyle & environment interacts with the genome to produce heritable changes resulting in phenotypic variation without even changing the DNA of the genome.

Epigenetic processes which include two changes i.e. DNA methylation and demethylation and post translational processes such as, acetylation phosphorylation and methylation of core histones, which result in an different histone code.

Epigenetic changes, which were well-described in the field of cancer, are now implicated in the pathogenesis of other diseases like obesity and insulin resistance. Epigenetic modifications have been described in various animal studies, although human study in light of epigenetics is difficult. This is due to the fact that human samples have been limited to blood cells while most of the epigenetic changes have been observed to be tissue-specific.

To stop the epidemic of rising chronic diseases, some the concept of FOAD is gaining much attention. The hypothesis proposed by David Barker has far-reaching implications as indicated by the following statement by the World Health Organization, "The global burden of death, disability and loss of human capital as a result of impaired fetal development is huge and affects both developed and developing countries." Intra-uterine environment is a delicate phase for the mother and for the offspring as well. As these broad and precise actions in the surrounding of pregnant female can affect "the product of conception" positively or negatively. These actions mainly include dietary, recreational, emotional etc.

Shadgarbhakara Bhava (six procreative factors) are not only the factors that are responsible for new progeny, but they are responsible for organogenesis and transferring other traits to the offspring. These traits are similar to the ones carried by chromosomes/genes as per modern concepts of embryogenesis, fetal growth, and development. Any changes in these traits may lead to certain diseases like Arbuda. As stated earlier, Arbuda or Cancer has emerged as second leading cause of death globally, there is need to emphasize on ancient saying- "Prevention is better than cure". Since environment plays a pivot role in prevalance of Arbuda, therefore it seems mandatory to provide the healthiest possible environment during the intrauterine period and after that as well. Pregnancy should be by choice not instance. Hence, proper mind makeup of the mother and ante-natal care is essential so that healthy genes are transmitted and the occurrence of dreadful disease like Arbuda can be prevented.

Epigenetics and Cancer Preventive Aspect

In scientific studies it has been seen that only 5–10% of all cancer cases can be caused due to genetic defects, the other 90–95% occur due to defect in the environment and lifestyle. The lifestyle factors include mainly any type of addiction like cigarette smoking, diet (fried foods, red meat), alcohol, sun exposure, environmental pollutants, infections, stress, obesity, and lack of exercise. As per the records it has been seen that all cancer-related deaths, almost 25–30% are due to tobacco, as many as 30–35% are linked to diet, about 15–20% are due to infections, and the remaining percentage are due to other factors like radiation, stress, physical activity, environmental pollutants etc .Therefore, cancer can be prevented by smoking cessation, increased ingestion of fruits and vegetables, moderate use of alcohol, caloric restriction, exercise, avoidance of direct exposure to sunlight, minimal meat consumption, use of whole grains, use of vaccinations, and regular check-ups.

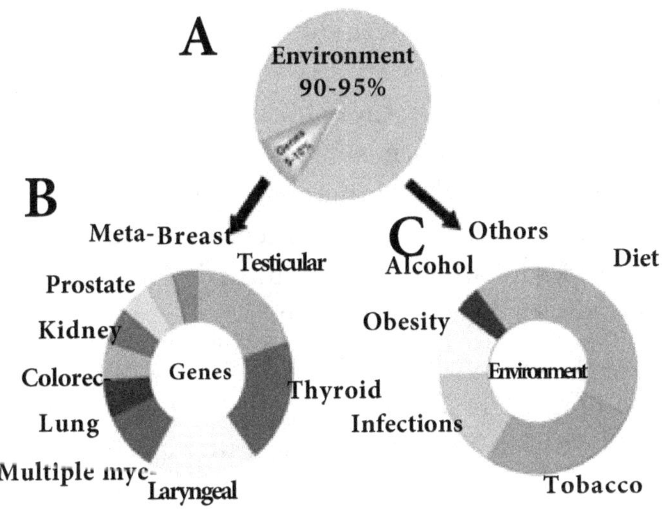

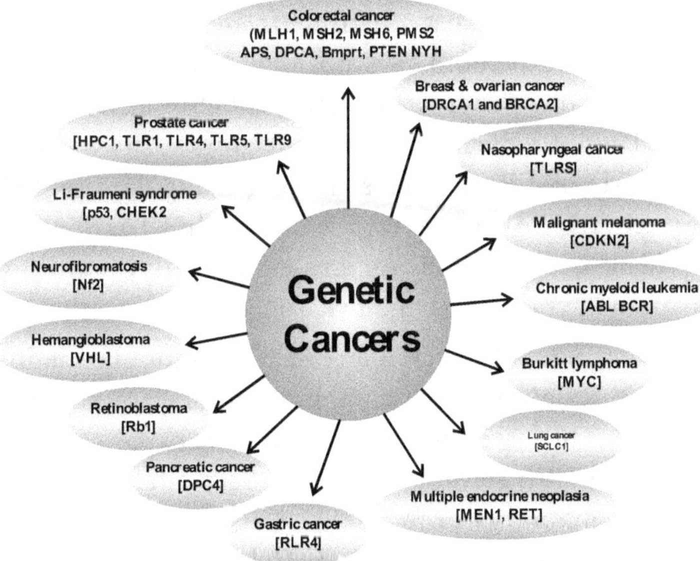

As mentioned earlier most cancers are not of hereditary origin and that lifestyle factors, such as dietary habits, smoking, alcohol consumption, and infections, have a great influence on their development. The science of epigenetics has explanation that how these dietary & lifestyle changes can bring changes in genetic expression. These factors have great impact on epigemone by loss of methylation affecting CpG sites (cytosine-phosphate-guanine) which were previously methylated. Due to the presence of these methyl groups a DNA conformation is there which blocks access to certain genes and renders them "silent". As many of genes are normally epigenetically silenced in every differentiated cell type, the unwanted activation of these genes due to de-methylation often increases unwanted gene expression.

Many studies suggest that DNA methylation and other persisting epigenetic changes to both DNA and chromatin induce differentiated direct cells back into a "stem-cell like" state predisposing to cancer, partly explaining a higher risk of carcinogenesis in older people or those chronically exposed to toxic agents. The dietary constituents, by affecting the DNA methylation status, bothways positively or negatively affect disease risk and progression and probably also the aging process. There are dietary enzyme co-factors such as folate and vitamins B12 and B6, as well as methyl group donors such as methionine, choline, betaine and serine that increase methylation, and selenium green tea polyphenols and bioflavonoids that reduce methylation.

It is a fact that the hereditary factors cannot be modified, but the lifestyle and environmental factors are potentially modifiable. The lesser hereditary influence of cancer and the capacity to modify nature of the environmental factors point to the preventability of cancer. The causative lifestyle factors that affect the incidence and mortality of cancer include tobacco, alcohol, diet, obesity, infectious agents, environmental pollutants, and radiation.

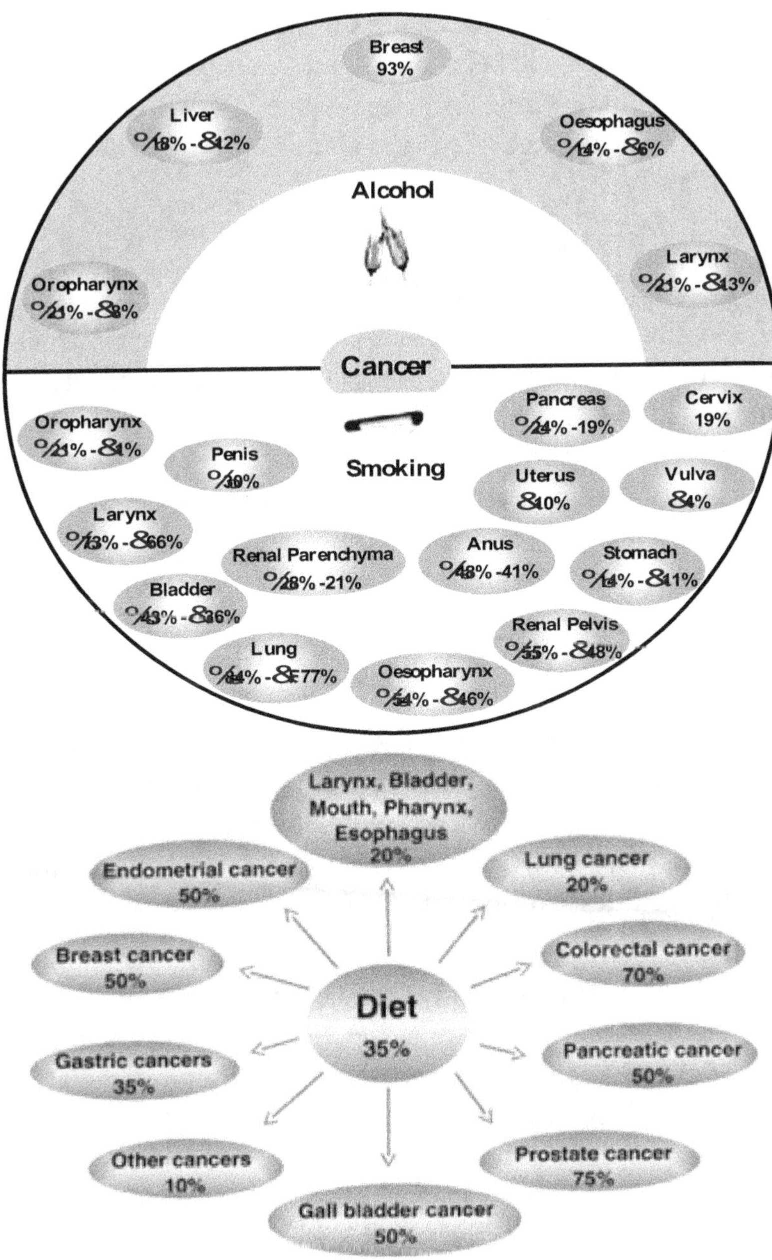

Ayurveda recommends a very unique and personalised approach to healthy eating which emphasizes freshness, moderation, variation and including the six tastes. Adequate cooking methods will help "pre-digest" most foods; about 20% of foods should be raw. Properly prepared, slowly eaten foods enjoyed in a relaxed setting will no doubt lead to better epigenetic health.

EPIGENETICS AND CANCER CURATIVE ASPECT

With the advancement of modern science, the treatment of acute diseases is possible due to the technical support. But the world is struggling with the burden of chronic lifestyle diseases due to poor diet and unhealthy lifestyle. Ayurveda which is time tested science treats the patient at personalised level while the modern medicine only treats the symptoms. In Ayurveda science the impact of mind is analysed on physical body while treatment of the person. In the science of epigenetics, this factor is not the genetic factor and it is possible to change it epigenetically which will positively or negatively effect the disease progress. According to classical literature the Caraka Samhita disease is initiated in the mind. The body and the mind cause a substrata of disease and happiness i.e. positive health. Balanced utilization of time, mental faculties, and object of sense organs is the cause of happiness.

Chronic inflammation is the key factor for causation of cancer. It is due to inflammation that is the risk of cancer increases. Any trauma or infection which causes inflammation is not directly linked with manifestation of neoplasia, it is the molecular mediators which were generated due to the process of inflammation. The key inflammatory factors like neutrophils, lymphocytes, monocytes, macrophages, and eosinophils generate the substances that are thought to mediate the development of inflammation-associated cancer, in this same process other cells also contribute, including the altered pre-cancerous cells themselves. Tumor necrosis factor, nitric oxide, adhesion molecules, derivatives of arachidonic acid (prostaglandins, leukotrienes), cytokines, chemokines, and free radicals are the inflammatory mediators responsible for manifestation of cancer. It is due to chronic exposure to these mediators which leads to increased cell proliferation, mutagenesis, modifications in epienome, activation of oncogene and the process of angiogenesis. The final step is the proliferation of cells that have run from normal growth control. Few scientific studies have revealed the evidences from animal models (i.e. mice, zebrafish) that cancer can be promoted due to chronic inflammation.

There is activation of inflammatory signal pathways such as the NF-κB signal pathway, signal transducer and activator of transcription 3 (STAT-3), and hypoxia-inducible factor 1alpha (HIF-1 alpha). Due to these there is release of release of inflammatory mediators such as the pro inflammatory cytokines (e.g. TNF and IL-1β) and pro inflammatory enzymes that are responsible for production of prostaglandins (e.g. COX-2) and leukotrienes (e.g. lipooxygenase), along with expression of adhesion molecules and matrix metalloprote-inases (MMPs). This process of events can lead to chronic inflammatory diseases such as arthritis, atherosclerosis, inflammatory bowel disease, chronic sinusitis, aging & cancer.

NF-κB (nuclear factor kappa-light-chain-enhancer of activated B cells) is a type of transcription factor central to the production of chronic inflammation. These transcription factors bind to regions of DNA just adjacent to the genes that they regulate. The transcription of the adjacent gene is either up- or down is regulated & depended on the transcription factor.

NF-κB is a protein complex that controls the transcription of DNA to messenger RNA, cytokine production and cell survival is dependent on the these factors. Scientists are trying to find that how these epigenetic modifications are passed on in cell division over many generations. It is not yet clear that although these modifications appear to be very stable, they can be modified by many factors including diet, chemicals, environment, pathological conditions, and even psychological state. Initiation is due to Inflammation and further development of cancer is depended upon the exposure to inflammation but the molecular mechanistic aspects of this phenomenon are not clearly understood. There is one model that links inflammation to the oncogenic transformation based on a positive feedback loop mechanism involving NF-κB, RNA-binding protein Lin-28, let-7 micro RNA, and IL-6 cytokine.

Clearly epigenetic factors play a crucial role in any such mechanism. in coming days under- standing and manipulating the epigenome, which is a potentially reversible source of biological variation, has great potential in chemopre- vention or stabilization of cancer. Now scientists are looking forward on modulating hyper/hypomethylation of key inflamma- tory genes influenced by dietary factors which will prove as an effective approach to cure or protect against cancer-inflam- mation.

- **The future of epigenetics is individualized therapies, the contemporary science may develop novel drugs with potential of targeting specific epigenetic components that has influenced by diet, lifestyle and the environment.**

- Future treatment may include drugs with epigenetic targets: DNA-MT inhibitors, HDAC inhibitors, etc.

References

- Cancer is a Preventable Disease that Requires Major Lifestyle Changes Preetha Anand,1 Ajaikumar B. Kunnumakara,1 Chitra Sundaram,1 Kuzhuvelil B. Harikumar,1 Sheeja T. Tharakan,1 Oiki S. Lai,1 Bokyung Sung,1 and Bharat B. Aggarwal1,2Pharmaceutical Research, Vol. 25, No. 9, September 2008.

- Binghamand S, Riboli E. Diet and cancer – the European prospective investi- gation into cancer and nutrition. Nat Rev Cancer 2004; 4:206–15.

- Anand P, Kunnumakkara AB, Sundaram C, Harikumar KB, Tharakan ST, Lai OS, et al. Cancer is a preventable disease that requires major lifestyle changes. Pharm Res 2008; 25:2097–116.

- Boffetta P, Couto E, Wichmann J, Ferrari P, Trichopoulos D, Bueno-de- Mesquita HB, et al. Fruit and vegetable intake and overall cancer risk in the European Prospective Investigation into Cancer and Nutrition (EPIC). J Natl Cancer Inst 2010; 102:529–37.

- Huang J, Plass C, Gerhauser C. Cancer chemoprevention by targeting the epigenome. Curr Drug Targets 2011; 12:1925– 56.

- Messinaand M, Hilakivi-Clarke L. Early intake appears to be the key to the proposed protective effects of soy intake against breast cancer. Nutr Cancer 2009; 61:792–8.

- [1]Sharma Annatram, Sushrut Samhita, 1stedi. Varanasi, Chaukhambha Subharti Prakashan, Sharirsthana 4/63pg. no. 62.

- [2]Sharma Annatram, Sushrut Samhita, 1st edi. Varanasi, Chaukhambha Subharti Prakashan, Sharirsthana 3/33 pg. no.43.

- Sharma Annatram, Sushrut Samhita, 1st edi. Varanasi, Chaukhambha Subharti Prakashan, Sharirsthana 3/33 pg.

no.43; Agnivesha. *Charaka* Samhita, Shrira sthana 3/24, edited & translated by Prof. Sharma PV. Chaukhambha orientalia. 9th ed. 2004. p. 424.

- Foetal Origin of Adult Disease; Kara Calkins, Sherin

- Pooja Sabharwal, Rima Dada, Chetan Prakash; Impact of Six Procreative Factors on Srotodushti of Garbha in Manifestation of FOAD (Foetal Origin of Adult Diseases).

- Foetal Origin of Adult Disease; Kara Calkins, Sherin

- Barker DJ. The developmental origins of adult disease. J Am Coll Nutr. 2004; 23:588S95S

- Kamini Dhiman, Abhimanyu Kumar, K S Dhiman; Shadgarbhkara Bhava vis-Œ-vis Congenital and Genetic Disorders.

- Foetal Origin of Adult Disease; Kara Calkins, Sherin

- Sharma Annatram, Sushrut Samhita, 1st edi. Varanasi, Chaukhambha Subharti Prakashan, Sutrasthana 24/7 pg. no.203.

- Sharma Annatram, Sushrut Samhita, 1st edi. Varanasi, Chaukhambha Subharti Prakashan, Sharirsthana 3/33 pg. no.43

- Sharma Annatram, Sushrut Samhita, 1st edi. Varanasi, Chaukhambha Subharti Prakashan, Sharirsthana 5/3(i) pg.no.69

- Sharma Annatram, Sushrut Samhita, 1st edi. Varanasi, Chaukhambha Subharti Prakashan, Sharirsthana 5/3(ii), (iii) pg.no.69

- Sharma Annatram, Sushrut Samhita, 1st edi. Varanasi, Chaukhambha Subharti Prakashan, Sharirsthana 3/18, 3/30 pg.no.35, 38

- Brahmanand Tripathi, Charak Samhita Purvardha, Varanasi, Chaukhambha Subharti Prakashan, Sharirsthana 4/9,10,11,16,20,21,22,23,24,25 pg.no. 878,885,886

•

5 Epigenetic Potential of Non Pharmacological Interventions

Cancer manifests due to emotional-psychic causes that sustained unresolved over long periods of time, and emotional healing and non pharmacological interventions provide the best cancer treatments. In humans there are maximum chances of development of different kind of lesions in different body parts & brain. Due to presence of such lesions there is formation of short circuit in the brain which if unresolved can give birth to cancerous tumours.

Illness occurs in the energy bodies surrounding our physical body on the consciousness level too. Due to the practice of adequate spiritual and emotional practices, these imbalances can be dissolved harmoniously. As severe negativity continuously generated in the energy bodies can eventually precipitate into the physical body causing various forms of pain and disease symptoms.

Chakras are energy circles in the body which are affected by the environment around. The positive or negative energy around the chakras decides the fate of health & disease. Manifestation of Cancer occurs near the most imbalanced chakra that is affected by a core issue in the body. Most of recent studies are changing that view and are increasingly establishing the connection between cancer and emotional trauma. Intervention of Ayurveda when one has cancer pain is very supportive way of treatment.

Cancer is a major public health problem in the US and many other countries of the world. Cancer is one of the leading causes of morbidity and mortality worldwide.

Cancer is the second dreadful barrier to increasing life expectancy in the 21st century. As per the report from the World Health Organization in 2015, cancer is the first or second leading cause of death before age 70 years in 91 of 172 countries, and it ranks third or fourth in an additional 22 countries. The report indicates that there will be 18.1 million new cases and 9.6 million cancer deaths worldwide.

Ayurveda has described cancer as "Vriddhi" or "*Arbuda*". As per the explanation, the blood becomes impure due to aggravation of one or more Dosha. This impurity of the blood is actually linked to *subtle* part of blood (*Rakta Dhatu*), and is not detected by physical tests. The impure blood along with aggravated *Dosha* circulated in the whole body and relocates in a region that has week immunity. Due to localization of improper *Rakta Dhatu*, *Prana* going the cells of that particular region also becomes impure. This is the reason of improper cell division.

Pain in cancer-

Pain has two dimensions-1. Unpleasant sensory (Physical), 2. Emotional experience (Psychological)

Pain is a multifaceted phenomenon that involves biological, psychological, and social consequences like as unrelieved severe pain may associated with disturbed sleep, reduced appetite, irritability and depression. Pain occur in estimates indicate that 50% of patients during process and in upto 75% of patients with advanced cancer. According to the International Association of Nurse in Cancer Care, 90% of pain could be treated with standard measure.

Observational data on the incidence of cancer pain survivalance indicate that a patients experience pain at some point during their course of treatment, and that pain impairs quality of life. In Cancer patients and survivors, the occurrence of pain firstly may raise concerns about disease progression and Second, biological factors e.g., tumor progression and invasion, or related treatments, it often persists after patients are believed to be cured of their cancer.

Usually the impact of psychological healing is underestimated by patients and health care professionals and they do not consider the potential benefits of using psychological treatments to manage cancer pain. This untreated pain leads to aggravation of the disease. Pain is one of the most feared and burdensome symptoms in cancer patients and often has a negative impact on patients functional status and quality of life. Supported attention to pain is the first priority to established quality improvement efforts. Being diagnosed and living with a life-threatening illness such as cancer is a stressful event that may affect of an individual's life.

Pain in patients with cancer is a stressful event which can affect patients life style also cause discomfort, loss of control, fatigue, and sexual activity, loss of interpersonal relationships and the concept of life, decreased performance, sleep and activities in them which has a negative impact on their healing process. Proper pain management may require a multidisciplinary approach.

Relation of Psychological Distress with pain-

Researchers have conducted various studies showing that there is a strong connection between cancer pain and psychological functioning. Some of the major findings of these studies are as follows:

These findings indicate that the cancer pain is linked to high levels of psychological distress, including higher levels of depression, anxiety, fear, and negative mood and fear of the future or pain progression. Effective relief of pain is depends upon a comprehensive assessment to identify physical, psychological, social, and spiritual aspects and multidisciplinary interventions. Careful assessment and management of psychological distress represents an important component in cancer pain management.

According to National Cancer Institute stress also can be lead to unhealthy behaviours, such as smocking or alcohol, that may affect cancer risk but can stress be a cause in and of itself. So along with herbal medicine patient will be treated with various unconventional therapies to control the defect in brain controlling mechanism.

Shad chakras-

The word *Chakra* literally means as wheel and a spinning sphere of energetic activity emanating from the major nerve ganglia branching of the spinal column. The *Chakras* are known to be a point or nexus of biophysical energy which are arranged along the spinal cord from bottom to top of the human body. The cerebrospinal system with nerve is the power house of the human body and the main switch in *Chakras*. Each *Chakra* is associated with certain alphabets called *Beeja Aksharas*, which need to be meditated to bring about balance of the *Chakras*.

	Chakras	Sthana	Elements	Vayu	Senses
1.	Muladhara chakra (Pelvic plexus)	Guda	Prithivi	Apana	Rasana
2.	Swadhishthan chakra (Hypogastric plexus)	Pedu	Jala	Vyana	Netra
3.	Manipura chakra (Coeliac plexus)	Nabhi	Agni	Samana	Twaka

4.	Anahata chakra (Cardiac plexus)	Hridaya	Vayu	Prana	Karna
5.	Vishuddha chakra	Kanth	Akash	Udana	
6.	Agya chakra	Bhrumadhya	Mahattatva		
7.	Sahasrara chakra				

Kundalini is the coiled serpent power, which is an enormous energy is locate at the base of the spine that is supposed to be awokened through the practice of meditation. According to ancient science *Prana* changes in consciousness, operate through the two canal of '*Ida* and *Pingala*' in humen being[9].

Epigenetic (Lifestyle) is a new biological field that is exploring the Effect of the environment on cells. The environment includes one's physical, social, and electromagnetic environment as well as confidence, awareness, lifestyle, habits, behaviors, and mind-body practices such as Pranic healing, plays a crucial role in affecting changes to our DNA. It is always wise to be surrounded by the positive environment as it has capability of changing the genetic expression.

Principles of Management in Ayurveda-

The living body is considered as amalgamation of earth, water, fire, air and space and they make not just the physical composition but also the mind and the soul[7]. So, the body as a whole includes mind, soul, behaviour and consciousness of an individual where the environment also plays a major role in making of a person.

The body is combination of *Sharir, Indriya, Satva, Aatma*. If any of these components are imbalanced or unconnected it can cause negative effect, such as disease. *Charaka Samhita* states that *Satva* or mind, *Aatma* or soul and

Sharira or body are just like the legs of tripod, on which the world rests[8]. Five elements combine with each other to give rise to three functional bio static energies (humour) of the body. These are responsible for all the physical, psychological function of body and mind.

Ayurvedic system is the first system to emphasize health as the perfect state of physical, psychological, spiritual component of Human being. It is important to maintain the strength of the patient during treatment. Cancer is not just a physical disease It is a disease of the mind and souls much as it is of the body.

The principle of Ayurveda believe that in the case of Cancer, the root cause may not necessarily be inside the body, factor could be the external factor. Cancer patients deal with various problems in different individual, family and social areas and also with the reduced life quality.

Nonpharmacologic interventions are important adjuncts to treatment modalities for patients with cancer pain. Various such kind of modalities can be used to reduce pain and concomitant mood disturbance and increase quality of life. Radiological, chemotherapy, hormones, and surgery all used to treat and palliate cancers, Combining these treatments with pharmacological and non-pharmacological methods of pain control. Cancer treatments, such as surgery, chemotherapy, radiation therapy, cause suffering and distress that lead to impaired quality of life for cancer survivors.

A combination of pharmacologic and non pharmacologic treatment modalities for cancer pain is the standard of care, as presented in World Health Organization guidelines.

Nonpharmacologic interventions are important supportive treatment modalities for patients with cancer pain. It can be used to reduce pain and concomitant mood disturbance and increase quality of life. In the classification of complementary medicine, energy healing class includes treatments in which the energy emanates from the human body (biofield) or is originated from an external source such as therapeutic touch, Reiki, shad chakras healing etc.

These Chakras are very important for energy balance and perfect synchronization of interior and exterior rythmus or HEF (Human Energy Field) and UEF (Universal Energy Field). Human beings are systems of energy and that the energy field is present a few inches beyond the skin's surface. Shadchakras energy healing process is a standardized biofield therapy that uses in the patient's "energy field" with the goal of restoring balance in the patient's energy system and strengthening the patient's "healing capacity" and to reduce distress and fatigue during chemotherapy.

Shadchakras energy healing process–

Scientific evidence provide tangible proof of the existence of body's energy and its relation to the health & well being. Pranic healing is an important component in the treatment of cancer .Stress can effect the *Aura*, causing gaps and interrupting Prana, the life-force. Clearing balancing and energizing the subtle body facilitates in restoring health.

Shad chakras have close relation with nervous system & collaboration with Yogic nadis *Ida, Pingala & Sushumna* and perform essential physical, mental and autonomus function. These *Nadis* are tubular organ of the body like an artery or vein and medium for flow of *Pranic* energy. Everyone practically experience various changes in the mental state like emotions, peaceful mind, excitation, remembrance etc. Due to dominance of *Ida- Pingala* activities.

In *Pranic healing exercise* both are equally flowing,

balanced, sympathetic and parasympathetic activities is established.

Chakras are the switches in path of energy flow, If these switches are off in normal person, they obstract the flow of energy, but when they are on, energy can ascend in *Susumna nadi.* A normal developed and opened *Chakras* always spins clockwise and gains *Pranic* energy from UEF while counter clockwise movement of a *Chakras* makes energy flow out which makes a *Chakra* closed, sick and abnormal.

The activities of the human body in the form of *Vayu.* *Pranavayu* flows continuously in *Ida, Pingala,* and *Sushumna* The energy is situated in *Muladhara chakra* called Kundalini shakti, it is the energy in static form & it is made kinetic by activating with meditation and spiritual practice and ascends in opened *Chakras* and reach to *Sahasrara* through these following processes-

1. Activation of the *Chakras*- Balancing and activating the chakras restores the natural healthy equilibrium of the body.divine spiritual energy run through the entire body, activating Chakras.

2. Treatment of the infection- the infection is treated from its roots. The immune system of the body is accelerated. Body's normal functioning is restored and any abnormality in the biological processes is resolved by divine spiritual energies.

3. Healing including regeneration of the cells and the damage caused by the infection or abnormality is treated. This final stage of healing oversees the complete renewal of the body's infected systems.

Each and every cell in the body requires the right quota of its *Prana* to carry on its biochemical processes in an efficient way. *Prana* is meta-physical energy that is responsible for living activities of human body. *Prana* can be described as vital energy that flows continuously inside the body and keeping human body alive. It is fire of life that manifests in the vitality.

Yogic texts have also explained that the energy back up required for live cellular activity is supplied from the six energy centres (Shad chakra). This *Prana* energy influences human's Neuro-hormonal system to balance hormonal profile and regulates different physiological functions in a living body. *Prana* influence our Central nervous system by acting on *Subtle* tasks such as perception, planning, execution, learning and memory. It increases alertness along with relaxation. *Prana* is sconcentrated in the *Shad-Charkas* and shows a reduction in sympathetic activity, it is key management of stress related disorders.

The aura has layers of physical, emotional, mental and spiritual elements. Yogic healing is an ancient spiritual skill achieved by the yogis through countless years of meditation & spiritual practice. The concept of body according to Tantra Shastra is the *Atisukshma* (finest) form.

Tantra shastra is the minutest and most powerful way of understanding the human body.

It focuses at the finest level of creation and deals mostly at the level of the mind, which is closest to the Atman. The language and expressions of tantric textbooks are filled with symbolizations, ritualism and has numerous esoteric meanings. The five *Mahabhoota*, mind and soul are represented in the form of seven energy centers in the central axis of the body.

The concept of *Chakra* have been used in the management of various disorders by means of *Daivavyapasraya* chikitsa and by means of various systems of sadhana. The seven Chakra respectively symbolizes the five *Mahabhoota*, the mind and the self, the seven levels of existence. The various letters of Sanskrit alphabet associated with the *Chakra* represent various frequencies of the matter energy wave which expresses itself as the world. The mastery over this is called as Mantra Shastra and the physical expression of these frequencies is known as Yantra Shastra.

The concept of a *Chakra* system of energy or consciousness centers exists in many forms in different indigenous systems including Egyptian, Chinese, Native American, Su, and Kabbalah.

Epigenetic potential of non pharmacological interventions.

According to Ayurvedic concepts each us of is born with a unique constitutional balance and the individual constitution or *Prakruti*, is based on physical and psychological characteristics (*Vata, Pitta, Kapha, Sattva, Raja, Tama*) and individual *Prakriti* roughly resembles our DNA, or our genes.

Epigenetic changes can also introduce for genetic instability and have a major role in the development of human cancer. In cancer survivals Radiations, Chemicals, Poor life style, Mental Stress, Oxidative stress cause disturbance the energy field (*Shadchakras*) and low immunity. These factors Disturbs the *Prakriti* (Genotype) (due to disturbance of (Phenotype) *Vata, Pitta, Kapha Satwa, Raja, Tama* that is DNA mutation which ultimately cause Cancer.

Alterations explained in epigenetics are induced by environmental stress associated with metabolic and neurodevelopmental disorders. Interestingly the epigenome has a reversible property since it is based on removable residues on genomic DNA. So, environmentally induced epigenomic alterations can be potentially restored. Here we discuss a specific therapeutic strategy based on the concept that a subtle, life-force energy pervades all living things. Balancing this proposed life-force energy is the goal of energy therapies.

Such interventions can help people relax and may improve quality of life. *Chakra* healing is a technique that aims to cleanse and balance the life-force energy in a person's body. This treatment can possibly be of great help in caring for cancer patients and reducing complications of the same. However, advanced studies are needed to evident the impact of *Shadchakras* healing with combination of contemporary measures.

Conclusion-

The study & knowledge of *Chakras*, *Chakra* energy balance and chakra healing are unconventional yet very friutful way of healing the body and mind and getting rid of many disease. Working on the *Chakras* on daily basis helps in living a healthy immune and disease free life.Ayurveda describe three modalities of treatment namely the *Daivavyapasraya*, *Yuktivyapasraya* and *Satvavajaya* into the nature of living systems. Based on this review, A statement can be made regarding the implication of *Shadchakra* healing as a non-invasive intervention like *Satvavajaya* chikitsa for improving the health status in patients with cancer.

It seems that this method can be used as a safe method in the management of physical function, pain, anxiety, depression and nausea in cancer patients and increasing a sense of well-being.

REFERENCE-

1. Global cancer statistics 2018: GLOBOCAN estimates of incidence and mortality worldwide for 36 cancers in 185 countries. Bray F, et al. citation-CA Cancer J Clin. 2018 Nov; 68(6):394-424. Doi: 10.3322/caac.21492. Epub 2018 Sep 12.

2. Sabharwal pooja, Spiritual healing for cancer through chakras. First Edition. Varanasi U.P. Chaukhamba Orientalia. 2009.

3. The International Association for the Study of Pain definition of pain: as valid in 2018 as in 1979, but in need of regularly updated footnotes. Pain Rep. 2018 Mar, 3(2): e 643. Published online 2018 Mar 5.

4. Jeannine M. Brant. The Global Experience of Cancer PAIN; Asian Pacific Journal of Cancer Prevention, Vol 11, 2010: MECC Supplement.

5. Elizabeth M. Thomas, PsyD, PhD, and Sharlene M. Weiss, RN, PhD. Nonpharmacological Interventions With Chronic Cancer Pain in Adult. March 1, 2000.

    http://doi.org/10.1177/107327480000700206

6. Dilip Kumar K.V. Clinical Yoga & Ayurveda. Chaukhamba Sanskit Pratisthan, Delhi. Edition 2011.P.114

7. Shukla V, Tripathi R, editors. Charaka Samhita Hindi Commentary Vol.2. First Edition. New Delhi: Chaukhamba Sanskrit Pratishthan; Reprint 2012.p. 750.

8. Shukla V, Tripathi R, editors. Charaka Samhita Hindi Commentary Vol.2. First Edition. New Delhi: Chaukhamba Sanskrit Pratishthan; Reprint 2012.p. 750.

9. Shastri Satynarayan. Charaka Samhita Hindi Commentary Vol.1 New Delhi: Chaukhamba Bharti Academy; Reprint 2012.p. 885.

10. Sabharwal Pooja. Discovery of the existence of human energy field (aura). unique journal of ayurvedic and herbal medicine. 2015 Mar 2; 62-3.

11. Sachin G. Khedikar, Avinash B. Chavan, Deepnarayan V. Shukla. Maintenance of sympathovagal balance in disease of Annavaha srotas through Yogic Nadis: A Review. Int. J. Res. Ayurveda Pharm. 2017; 8(1):4-7 http://dx.doi.org/10.7897/2277-4343.0812

12. Gherand Samhita. Shree pitambara peeth sanskrita parishad, M.P. Edition- 4, 13 july 2003.

13. Sabharwal Pooja. Effect of intervention of ayurveda & practical implementation of Shadchakras an indigenous approach as co- therapy with chemotherapy & radiotherapy for physical & mental well being of cancer patient. Journal of Ayurveda. 2 (Oct-Dec 2008); 28-33.

14. Dr. Rakesh Narayan V., Dr. Ashwathy kutty V.; A Study of Yogic and Vedic Anatomy in the perspective of Shadchakra. World Journal of Pharmaceutical Science; Vol.5 Issue 8,373-378.

15. K. Candis Best. A Chakra System Model of Lifespan Development. International Journal of Transpersonal Studies 29(2):112-118. July 2010.

●

6. Ayurveda and Metabolic Diseases in Purview of Epigenetics

Epigenetics is the contemporary science which deals with the study of cellular and physiological traits that are heritable by daughter cells without changes in the DNA sequence. There are some epigenetic processes like paramutation, bookmarking, imprinting, gene silencing, X chromosome inactivation, position effect, reprogramming, transection, maternal effects. These specific processes have their impact on phenotypic changes during foetal life. Most of the diseases have been seen caused by epigenetics now a days. Certain factors which influence epigenetic changes are exercise, drugs, Diet, addiction of Alcohol, environmental factors like Chemicals in the living space or workplace, any kind of Medications and many other unknown factors are linked to epigenetically changes. Despite the advancements in diagnostic techniques and therapeutic interventions, medical science has failed to keep the incidence of congenital malformations and metabolic disorders under control. Diseases explained in Ayurveda like factors responsible for them are now explainable in the language of epigenetics. Ayurveda principals can be applied to prevent and cure all those metabolic diseases which are caused in foetal life due to intrauterine changes due to epigenetic changes. The maternal and nutritional factors play a crucial role & physical, mental, social, and spiritual well-being of the person, and practice of a wholesome regimen, play a major role in achieving a healthy offspring and prevent metabolic disorders, thus building a healthy family, society, and nation.

- https://flipper.diff.org/app/pathways/info/723
- https://www.researchgate.net/publication/315807830 _ENLI GHTNING_EPIGENETICS_THROUGH_ AYURVEDA_AND_IT'S_ROLE_IN_FUTURE
- https://www.researchgate.net/publication/303323450_ Ayurvedic_Perspective_of_Pregnancy_and_Fetal_ Development_ During_the_First_and_Second_Trimester

•

7. Ayurveda as Preventive, Predictive and Personalized Medicine in Purview of Epigenetics and Oncology

Preventive, Predictive and Personalized Medicine in purview of Epigenetics and Oncology

One of the major contributors to the incidence of cancer is lifestyle. The higher incidence of cancer is found among immigrants from the Eastern world to the Western world. It further emphasizes the role of lifestyle. Conventional medicine has made some major strides in understanding cancer and its molecular basis, the knowledge about how to prevent or treat cancer is still aging behind.

A gene that predisposes us to a disease such as cancer, diabetes, Parkinson's, Grave's disease, etc might be present in us. In spite of this there is power to turn the expression of these 'bad' genes off through nutrition and lifestyle choices. Today's world contains many opportunities for becoming toxic which affects the human being at the molecular level ultimately causing changes in the gene expression.

Toxicity comes from many sources: our environment, food, water, skin products, cleaning products, radiation, heavy metals, and most mainly from our physic. Epigenetics is related to methylation. When this MTFR is defective it can increase your risk of various forms of cancer.

Ayurveda which is has been around for thousands of years, this science has always emphasized that lifestyle and environment are the keys to health and prevention of disease! The science of Ayurveda is all about prevention so that those bad genes could not express themselves. Ayurveda learning's also teaches how to get rid of disease once it is manifested in body. This way epigenetically we can predict, prevent and give personalized medicine to cancer patients.

Ayurveda teaches how to eat according to the constitution for optimal digestive health and wellbeing; it teaches us to keep a daily routine; to eat according to ritu (season); to get proper sleep; to maintain good personal hygiene; to participate in seasonal or routine detoxification, and so much more.

The incidences of cancer has increased year by year, a number of casualties occur due to it. and cancer is the second dreadful disease after cardiovascular diseases. It has been shown in many studies that tumor is a chronic disease involving the whole body.

The growth of tumors is involved in many stages and complex processes, and in many genes and molecular events including multi-gene mutations, such as activation of oncogenes and inactivation of tumor suppressor genes. A typical cancer occurrence model needs the mutation of two to eight driver genes.

The mutation of only passenger genes is not able to lead the development of cancer. It depends on the central dogma; mutation in the gene pattern may affect a series of mRNA and protein expressions.

Along with the development of cancer biomarkers, it has been found in studies that the change of key molecule panel in gene and protein sequences initiates the tumor genesis. Because different individual has different key molecule panel. Recently, many patients are putting attentions on precision therapy, which needs more and more biomarkers to be found.

The best optimal biomarker is only changes in cancer patients and can be easily detected. The most common cancer biomarkers are generally to detect the removed cancer tissues, which is an invasive operation. The growth of cancer is a complicate progress. Different forms from DNA, RNA, protein to metabolite, all the differences in the levels of DNA, RNA, protein, and metabolite between cancer patients and health persons could be called biomarkers. Less invasive, early and effective biomarkers are still limited, although many biomarkers have been found. The biomarkers that are used are from the four ways: (i) metabolic products of tumor cells, (ii) abnormal differentiation of cellular gene products, (iii) tumor necrosis and exfoliation of tumor cells release into the blood circulation, and (iv)cell reactive products of tumor host cells. These biomarkers can be detected when cancer occurred. Before cancer occurred, DNA/RNA/protein and the environment changes in normal cells could make normal cell changes into differentiation disorder cell, which is known cause of cancer. With the advancement of image technology, it was founded that imaging features of cancer appearance have a close relationship with the diagnosis and prognosis of patients.

Imaging features is becoming a new type of biomarkers. Biomarkers can be divided into two categories: (i) contribution to the mechanism and therapeutic targets, and (ii) contribution to prediction, diagnostic test, and prognosis assessment. The pathogenesis of the disease has direct relationship with the biomarker which is further linked with occurrence of disease.

The early detection of the type of biomarkers is needful before occurrence of the disease. The biomarkers are not required to change. There is specific pattern of biomarkers. It is easy to treat cancer after pattern recognition which recognizes pattern biomarker for specificity of prediction, diagnosis, prognosis, and prevention/therapy of tumor.

P3 medicine in cancer

In humans it has been seen that the most complicated and diverse phenotypic traits relative to any other living organisms are present. Various studies predict that only 0.1% of the entire genome differs between individuals. The genomic diversities are affected by many ethnic and geographic differences in a wide variety of traits. The high rate of heritable mutations and subtle variants contribute to somatic alterations.

All of those lead to cellular traits that aggravate carcinogenesis, which determines individual's risk to develop certain cancers. There is a prime role of cancer biomarkers in proliferation, invasion, and metastasis, and are related to prevention, diagnosis, and treatment including acquired drug resistance. Therefore, in conventional oncology, the most important goal is to find the ways to effectively control tumor heterogeneity and translate these achievements to benefit patients.

Proper clinical trial allocation has been based on the right target, right drug, and right moment, so most trials focus on those patients who share the similar targetable biomarkers. Although cells within tumors have diverse genomes and epi genomes, and interact differentially with their surrounding microenvironment that includes extracellular matrix, inflammatory cells, immune cells, endothelial cells, fibroblasts, etc.

Collectively those factors generate intra-tumor heterogeneity, which has critical implications for treating cancer patients. Therefore it is a challenge of tumor diversity for managing the treatment of cancer patients.

Taking the knowledge of whole-genome, whole-exome, and whole transcriptome sequencing offer an appropriate approach and opportunities for discovery, but their immediate effect on clinical decision-making is still limited. The most important goal for scientific community is to find the ways to effectively control tumor heterogeneity and translate these achievements to benefit patients. The development of cancer is a complex process and affected by many factors, that is why a single biomarker that resolves the relative problems of a cancer is false information.

The incidence of cancer has increased gradually and the casualties due to cancer has raised. Due to early treatment survival rate can be increased many folds. The gene pattern derived from high-risk group can be used to perform risk assessment, and improve cancer screening, early diagnosis, and treatment.

Because of the tumor heterogeneity, gene mutations differ in different patients. Which lead to different sensitivity to the drug. So identity the differentially expressed genes was needed for precise treatment. In the process of cancer treatment some effective cancer biomarkers have been discovered and used in clinic practice. However, due to low specificity of these proteins, it only plays a supporting role, but not a determining factor in clinic diagnosis. With further studies, more and more differentially expressed proteins or peptides will be found; these proteins or peptides combined to form a pattern, increases pecificity of the tumor diagnosis, and reduce the false positive rate.

Chronic diseases, otherwise known as non communicable diseases (NCDs), represent the major global health problem of the 21st century. The major chronic diseases listed by World Health Organization (WHO) are cardiovascular disease (CVD), cancer, chronic respiratory diseases and diabetes mellitus (DM); neurodegenerative disorders are also a significant concern.

Chronic diseases are the world's leading cause of health burden and mortality and are continuing to increase in both incidence and prevalence. Chronic diseases are a major cause of poverty and obstruct economic development. The chronic disease has some common risks including socio-economic factors, cluster in co-morbidities. The most important challenge for chronic diseases in the 21st century is to deal with their complexity and the often 'silent' transition from health to disease with a late onset of symptoms which can delay treatment and interventions and to shift towards prevention.

Fortunately, the majority of chronic diseases can be prevented or delayed until significantly later in life through interventions such as adoption of a healthy lifestyle throughout the lifespan resulting in an extended health span. Balancing normal values for key health metrics, such as blood pressure (BP), lipids, and blood glucose also play a primary role in reducing chronic disease risk.

Proper understanding of genomics and the interaction between genomics, lifestyle, personal experiences of adversity and the social and physical environment, the possibility to predict risk and prevent chronic disease will be further improved.

However, a new healthcare delivery system is needed to implement these mechanisms properly. For example, Halfon and Hochstein introduced the Life Course Health Development (LCHD) concept that describes "how health trajectories develop over an individual's lifetime due to positive and negative experiences and how this knowledge can guide new approaches to policy and research." It is becoming much clearer that early life adversity from poverty, abuse and neglect has long lasting influences on health and contributes disproportionately to the health care burden.

The current framework of healthcare and chronic disease management is largely ineffective. There is a need to re think about the paradigm shift to focus on wellness and the prevention of chronic disease and associated risk factors first and foremost.

The concept of wellness, an optimal state of health, is a new concept for transforming healthcare. The healthcare must shift its focus to promoting a state of wellness, from the individual to population level in future. Also following wellness to disease transitions and learning how to reverse common diseases at their earliest possible stage.

Within the coming years, we predict that the ability to better define true human wellness will be further refined through advancements in numerous scientific fields including blood biomarkers. In instances where risk factors or an actual chronic disease diagnosis has manifested, the focus must shift to aggressively return an individual to a state of health and wellness. Moreover, there is wide agreement that the stakeholders involved and the interventions and programming needed to combat chronic disease must expand and embrace a multi sector approach. Clearly, the reactive health care model that currently exists is suboptimal, requiring a paradigm shift to improve global to individual health and address the current challenges we face with chronic disease and associated risk factors. We need a new approach, focusing on care that is preventive, predictive and personalized or (P3) medical concept as core principles of the continuum model.

Predictive:

The prediction of dysfunctions and detecting disease pre-cursors at Stage B provide opportunity for early interventions to combat the underlying mechanisms before symptoms occur. The predictive medicine is essential for the preventive medicine.

The application of predictive medicine at early stage requires active role of health care professionals in addressing and interacting with 'healthy individuals,' without signs or symptoms, to detect the early risk of emerging dysfunctions, for preventing a progression in stage of health at a minimum and ideally facilitating a regression to stage A.

A biomarker is actually an indicator of a biological state of human being also the past or present existence of a particular type of organism. It is not actually a genomic or post-genomic one. for many diseases like cancer, clinically useful biomarkers are just beginning to appear and are not yet wide spread. The future systems biology research will help to explore new biomolecular networks and biomarkers for disease prediction and monitoring.

For pharmacogenomics the biomarkers and targets will also be of interest to improve bio-pharmaceutical interventions. At present the 'classic biomarkers' such as blood lipids, blood glucose and C-reactive protein are at the core of predicting diseases. More & more research of biomarkers will increase the precision of identifying dysfunctions, ideally early in the process.

Preventive:

Preventing chronic disease is the preferred approach for moving forward towards disease free nation. There is decline in functional and physiologic health parallel with advancing age and/or manifestation of chronic disease and co-morbidity. The process of aging is associated with, chronic diseases and co-morbidities, thereby marking their effects on health and well-being.

While moving from stage A to stage B the quality of life, autonomy and life expectancy are greatly reduced. The preventive apparoach can be applied to reduce the decline in functional and physiologic health. Preventing diseases as early as possible requires a proper understanding of chronic disease pathogenesis, which comes from implementing systems medicine approaches that identify relevant disease related networks, and the influence of risk factors as well as potential protective factors. Preventing disease in Stage A ensures risk factors for chronic disease never manifest & that is known as primordial prevention.

Personalized:

The current conventional medicine has made guidelines regarding the individual receiving care without an appreciation of the complexities of human biology and its unique interaction with the surrounding environment. This approach has led to suboptimal outcomes for a large percentage of individuals receiving care. Research is going on to illustrate the importance of personalized medicine.

For example, research in the area of personalized nutrition has revealed highly inter-individual responses to standardized meals, highlighting the importance of not taking a one-size-fits-all approach. As the response to physical exercise and psychological stress is also highly variable and depends on genetic profiles of individuals and lifestyles. It has been seen that the chronic disease risk in general has a genetic component. The approach to chronic diseases like cancer is already moving towards a more personalized approach based on individual phenotyping and molecular targeting.

Stages of health

The chronic disease manifestation and the transition from health to a chronic disease can be divided into four primary stages. This explanation is based on the model of allostasis and allostatic load and overload. Allostasis is the active process of adaptation to daily experiences, may be good or bad, and allostatic load and overload refer to the cumulative change in the entire system of the brain and body. When it is experienced by human being the "toxic stress" created inside effects both psychologically and physiologically leads to disease. These negative health behaviors related to a stressful lifestyle contribute to allostatic load and overload.

In this process, initially, an individual moves from health, Stage A, to noticeable signs, or biological expression, in stage B, where early disease precursors and dysfunctions can be detected but the individual is unaware of them and does not have any symptoms, which is common in clinical medicine. Further chronic diseases usually progress slowly, the individual showing symptoms, and clinical expression is the Stage C at this point at which conventional reactive health care is initiated.

Although advancements in interventions are there even though many individuals with symptoms will make the transition to confirmed chronic disease, Stage D, where conventional healthcare and other interventions used to manage the chronic disease. After reaching Stage D and a chronic disease diagnosis is confirmed, there is permanent physiologic damage/dysfunction is there.

Let's take few examples, in ischemic damage after a myocardial infarction or stroke, cancer and other chronic diseases will leave permanent damage and dysfunctions. In the current health care system, such kind of damage usually requires lifelong treatment and management. Despite of this the individuals who are keen to improve core components of their health, has the potential to significantly improve their prognosis, clinical status and quality of life.

Stage A: Apparently healthy and avoiding the accumulation of stressors

Stage A indicates an individual is in apparently good health and wellness. Individuals in Stage A indicate healthy lifestyle characteristics like regular physical activity, no addiction, healthy diet, and holds key health measures within the normal range like blood glucose, BP, blood lipids. At this stage the individuals are able to adapt the potential threats to their survival and changes in their environment in order to maintain homeostasis and promote survival.

The term 'apparently' healthy is coined because at this time there is no tool available to determine levels of poor health beyond the presence of clinical risk factors. Although even in absence of biomarkers research is in progress for identifying more granular risk categories. For general public such genomics and other detailed biological, clinical, environmental and molecular assessments are currently not readily available for assessment. After performing detailed molecular assessments for a larger percentage of the population, the characterization and definition of apparent health in Stage A will become refined and more precise. Already progress in this direction has begun with precision medicine initiatives. Large, dense, dynamic, personalized data collection, such as the one being generated by the 100 K wellness project, are specific examples of a movement towards precision medicine.

These efforts are creating the framework for "scientific wellness," where millions of data points, from DNA, blood, saliva, the micro biome and lifestyle, among others, will be used to exponentially refine how an individual's health is managed and optimized.

It's a hard & annoying fact that those who possess Stage A health comprise a very small percentage of the current global population. In addition to this, most individuals are scattered in a world that is far from what can be characterized as health-promoting. So, this poor health environment which has limited access to nutritious food, a physically inactive environment and limited effective social network interactions, etc. is a communicable condition.

It can be said that the poor health characteristics of an environment can be transmitted to an individual. The human being thus has created a world where the ability of an individual to remain in Stage A is increasingly difficult. A global health goal must be directed towards substantially increasing the percentage of the population that remains in Stage A health, providing an inoculation from unhealthy environments.

The cause of chronic diseases shares a common cluster of environmental and lifestyle risk factors or stressors like physical inactivity, poor nutrition, psychosocial distress, excess body mass, indoor and outdoor air and sound pollution, tobacco, inadequate sleep, excess stress, etc. Similarly socio-economic determinants, especially poverty, also influence the generation, severity and management of chronic diseases. It is due to the constant exposure to these stressors and poor health behaviors that are responsible for the journey towards allostatic overload and resulting chronic disease.

Stress factors or distress, are complexly associated with sustained local and systemic inflammation as well as a host of other dysfunctions. These stressors can even start early in life reflecting effects of abuse, neglect and poverty, with significant negative health implications during adulthood that contribute disproportionately to the healthcare burden. For example children exposed to adverse childhood experiences like psychosocial, socioeconomic disadvantage, maltreatment and social isolation are at increased risk for depression, increased systemic inflammation and clustered metabolic derangements in adulthood.

The cause of a complex set of disorders such as chronic diseases cannot be pin-pointed to a single origin, it is actually a highly complex interacting network of many mediators and factors that interact on different levels over time and space is involved. It is also important to note that biological systems work in a non-linear way, with the brain as the central organ of adaptation or mal-adaptation. Some factors can increase resilience against stressors and maintain an individual in Stage A; like healthy nutrition and physical activity can reduce the risk of cancer and CVD; healing practices can modulate interception to attenuate affective and psychosomatic disorders and reduce perceived stress and neurogenic inflammatory response. Meaning and purpose in life and social connectedness also promote better health.

Interestingly, telomeres provide an example of how these factors can impact the rate of biological aging even in the absence of disease. Most of these positive lifestyle resiliency factors have been related to longer telomere length. Further, a positive lifestyle appears to protect telomere shortening when under psychological stress.

Such kind of preventive activities can be effectively personalized to the individual e.g., providing feedback through monitoring. Along with a healthy lifestyle, there is lot of work to be done with how pharmaceutical or other interventions could potentially increase resilience towards outside stressors and prevent diseases. It is actually a interesting fact that a certain amount of positive stress (i.e., eustress) is necessary to maintain health; physical exercise and caloric reduction result in eustress, leading to positive biological adaptations.

Moving from Stage A (i.e., allostasis) to the beginning of a pre-chronic disease, Stage B (i.e., allostatic load), is usually of slow progression and often unnoticed by the individual undergoing this transition.

Stage B: The chronic disease signs appearance

The intertwined multitude of stressors most individuals are exposed to in Stage A lead to complex phenotypes that eventually manifest as clinical and biologic signs. The stage B of the disease actually marks the initiation of noticeable process associated with increased chronic disease risk. The signs include elevated BP, dyslipidemia, and elevated blood glucose. Measures of chronic inflammation have emerged as important signs for chronic disease risk and it has predictive value for later disease.

Recently the science of genomics, epigenetics, trans-criptomics, proteomics, metabolomics and gut micro biome are analyzing the relation to chronic disease risk prediction to evolve the future discovery which will refine the identification of individuals in Stage B with these parameters. The 'omics' are usually thought of as providing a disease signature but they are even more valuable in the transition from Stage A to Stage B.

Many factors like excess body mass, mostly the visceral fat, is also a significant predictor of chronic disease risk and associated adverse events. Similarly exercise performance and body habitus, while recognized as important markers of health and prognosis, are actually not viewed as "signs" of chronic disease risk. There is a paradigm shift in this mindset and accordingly the below-normal exercise performance and excess body mass be treated as signs of increased chronic disease risk and represent an individual to be classified as Stage B.

Early dysfunctions and chronic disease pre-cursors as signs of allostatic load are often overlooked in the traditional health care setting. Individuals with the classic initial signs of chronic disease risk such as high BP, blood glucose and dyslipidemia as well as recently discovered signs such as telomere length shortening and changes in the gut micro-biome usually do not go along with functional impairment in daily life.

The diminished exercise performance is also usually undetected in the general population. This lack in exercise is due to the fact that a big percentage of the population, particularly those at greatest risk for one or more chronic diseases, leads a sedentary lifestyle, avoiding levels of exertion that would likely manifest an exertional Stage B sign.

Mostly the individuals are unaware of their increased movement from health towards a chronic disease or they are not willing to take steps to reverse this process, they are not ready to take preventive, proactive measures, such as lifestyle modifications or biological or pharmaceutical interventions. These days the current efforts seek to empower individuals with knowledge to optimize wellness and reverse this process of disease. It is utmost important to intervene this educational approach to science education. It is very helpful to view this early health monitoring, psychological education, and counseling. The knowledge and motivation can immunize young people from continuing down the silent path of chronic disease.

Stage C:

In today's traditional reactive healthcare system, the manifestation of chronic disease symptoms is a common entry point for individuals like in dyspnea which is occurring within the range of exertional capacity needed for activities of daily living is a Stage C symptom. Constant depression should also be viewed as a symptom that elevates chronic disease risk. Significant pathophysiologic dysfunction is well established in this stage. Unhealthy lifestyle characteristics and abnormalities in key health measures are, in the vast majority of cases, also well established in Stage C and now compounded by outwardly apparent symptoms. In the contemporary healthcare system, the symptoms are oftentimes treated without addressing the poorly understood underlying causes and mechanisms that are at the root of the dysfunction, which are in large part unhealthy lifestyle behaviors. Symptoms become temporarily aggravated as the level of dysfunction persists and progressively worsens as do the unhealthy lifestyle behaviors, giving rise to subsequent symptomatic episodes and progressive biological damage. At this phase, the risk for the diagnosis of a chronic disease and conversion to Stage D is high.

Stage D: Final stage of confirmed chronic disease diagnosis

When the chronic disease is diagnosed the treatment approach is more aggressive and this is the stage of defining moment of the reactive health care model. To treat chronic disease, such as coronary artery disease or cancer, requires expensive and often invasive interventions. It differs from Stage C as in that case the underlying causes and mechanisms of the diagnosed chronic disease are not addressed. The active health care model is focused on stabilizing the individual in a hospital setting and ameliorating acutely elevated symptoms.

Environmental and lifestyle risk factors are usually not addressed at this stage even, which if modified substantially improve prognosis and quality of life. As a result of this dysfunction continues and symptoms worsen with morbidity and premature mortality and increasing health care costs as the end result.

Health stages

Health Stages which have been described earlier from A–D should not be viewed as unidirectional or stationary, progressing from apparent health to chronic disease with no ray of hope of reversal. A good storehouse of information clearly demonstrates improving health behaviors and key health metrics significantly improve an individual's future health trajectory. An individual who has been diagnosed with a chronic disease may ameliorate all Stage C symptoms and Stage B signs by improving health metrics and lifestyle behaviors.

Integration of principles

P3 medicine & other systems medicine, considers human biological systems as a cohesive whole. Eastern medicine also considers the human body as a holistic entity of harmonious organs and approaches health from this framework. These principles are mainly derived from Chinese and Indian cultures, with long-term practical experience in the prevention, diagnosis and treatment of chronic diseases.

Ayurveda and P3 medicine & epigenetics

Ayurveda is an ancient wisdom of personalized medicine documented and practiced in India since 1500 B. C. In this present era, Ayurveda not only plays a key role in Indian health care systems but is also increasingly recognized in the whole world health model. In Ayurveda there is the deep understanding of the biological basis of human individuality through Prakriti (literally meaning basic nature or the healthy state which can be considered as Stage A. According to Ayurveda, an individual is born with a specific Prakriti that not only determines an individual's overall phenotype but also predicts the susceptibility to diseases and his reaction to extrinsic and intrinsic environments.

Assessment of the disease state which is known as vikriti and treatment in the Ayurveda system depend on "where you were and where you are now" with respect to an individual's own Prakriti and how much influence on specific Dosha has occurred to create imbalance leading to a state of Vikriti that is Stages B–D. Ayurvedic medicine treats holistically in combination of medicine, diet and lifestyle management with the ultimate goal of returning to one's original state of Prakriti. In recent years, many efforts have been initiated in to establish the molecular correlation with specific Prakriti. These efforts in translating the concepts of P3 medicine and establishing the relationship of phenotypic classification of Ayurveda with contemporary genomic analysis has led to the convergence of two disciplines and emergence of the new field of Ayurgenomics & epigenetics. Various studies, efforts are being made to correlate differences in epigenetic markers (DNA methylation) with various Prakriti phenotypes along with Genome-Wide SNP Analysis as correlates of Ayurveda Prakriti.

References

- Akesson A, Larsson SC, Discacciati A, Wolk A. Low-risk diet and lifestyle habits in the primary prevention of myocardial infarction in men: a populationbased prospective cohort study. J Am Coll Cardiol. 2014; 64:1299–1306.

- Shonkoff JP, Boyce WT, McEwen BS. Neuroscience, molecular biology, and the childhood roots of health disparities: building a new framework for health promotion and disease prevention. JAMA. 2009;301:2252–2259.

- An Observational Study for Assessment of Dehaprakriti in Mamsarbuda (Myoma) in Predictive, Preventive and Personalized Medical Concept.

- Michael Sagnera. The P4 Health Spectrum – A Predictive, Preventive, Personalized and Participatory Continuum for Promoting Healthspan. Progress in Preventive Medicine. 2017; 1-13, DOI: 10.1097/pp9.00000000000000002.

- McEwen BS. Protective and damaging effects of stress mediators. New Engl J Med. 1998;338:171–179.

- Peters A, McEwen BS. Editorial introduction. Physiol Behav. 2012;106:1–4.

- Hood L, Price ND. Demystifying disease, democratizing health care. Sci Transl Med. 2014;6:225ed5, http://dx.doi.org/10.1126/scitranslmed.3008665.

- Hood L, Price ND. Promoting wellness and demystifying disease: the 100K project. Clin Omics. 2014;1:20–21.

- Jackson SE, Steptoe A, Wardle J. The influence of partner's behavior on health behavior change: the English Longitudinal Study of Ageing. JAMA Intern Med. 2015;175:385–392.

- Auffray C, Chen Z, Hood L. Systems medicine: the future of medical genomics and healthcare. Genome Med. 2009;1: 1–11.

- Michael Sagnera. The P4 Health Spectrum – A Predictive, Preventive, Personalized and Participatory Continuum for Promoting Healthspan. Progress in Preventive Medicine. 2017; 1-13, DOI: 10.1097/pp9.0000000000000002.

- Niiranen TJ, Vasan RS. Epidemiology of cardiovascular disease: recent novel outlooks on risk factors and clinical approaches. Expert Rev Cardiovasc Ther. 2016;14:855–869, http://dx.doi.org/10.1080/14779072.2016.1176528. [Epub 2016 Apr 25].

- Crump C, Sundquist J, Winkle by MA, Sundquist K. Interactive effects of physical fitness and body mass index on the risk of hypertension. JAMA Intern Med. 2016; 176:210–216.

- An Observational Study for Assessment of Dehaprakriti in Mamsarbuda (Myoma) in Predictive, Preventive and Personalized Medical Concept.

- Twig G, Yaniv G, Levine H, et al. Body-mass index in 2.3 million adolescents and cardiovascular death in adulthood. N Engl J Med. 2016;374:2430–2440, http://dx.doi.org/10.1056/NEJMoa1503840. [Epub 2016 Apr 13].

- Trefois C, Antony PM, Goncalves J, Skupin A, Balling R. Critical transitions in chronic disease: transferring concepts from ecology to systems medicine. Curr Opin Biotechnol. 2015;34:48–55.

- Michael Sagnera. The P4 Health Spectrum – A Predictive, Preventive, Personalized and Participatory Continuum for Promoting Healthspan. Progress in Preventive Medicine. 2017; 1-13, DOI: 10.1097/pp9.

8 Epigenetics & Ayurveda in Healthy Aging

Ayurveda as bioenergetic medicine in healthy aging in purview of epigenetics

In Ayurveda, living body is considered as combination of earth, water, fire, air and space which makes the physical and mental constitution of the human body. The history of this science is extensive—extending back thousands of years. Many years ago, ancient tradition of India mentioned about a universal energy called prana. This universal energy is the source of all life activities.

That is, the body as a whole includes mind, soul, behaviour and consciousness of an individual where the environment also plays a major contribution in making of a person. In modern anatomy human body is made up of systems, tissues and cells from gross to subtle level.

Scientific evidence provide tangible proof of the existence of body's energy and its relation to the health & well being. Bio energetic medicine is the branch of science which deals with the treatment of subtle & cosmic body and deals with healing through five senses, meridians, chakras and energy healing.

There is clear mention of treating Prana (bioplasmic body) in ancient science. Epigenetics is a branch of biology that is examining the effect of the environment on cellular behaviour. The "environment" means one's physical, social, and electromagnetic environment as well as all beliefs, perceptions, lifestyle, habits, behaviours, and mind-body practices such as Pranic healing.

As per the concept of epigenetics mapping of genes is possible that keep us in a healthy state and eliminate those bad genes that have been plaguing humans over the course of time. Although advancement is there in public health and medical care, the ten leading causes of death for persons over age 65 have not changed appreciably in the past several decades. Also the rank order of mortality causes has remained essentially the same. In coming years the proportion of elderly is expected to grow to 22%. The elderly population is becoming older also. At present 12% of the elderly population are the "oldest old" or aged 85 or older. Most important target is to claim the physical, emotional, mental layer of body system. Several clinical conditions and diseases which commonly afflict the aged have been studied with Ayurveda as bioenergetic medicine in purview of epigenetics.

The main diseases that increase in frequency and severity with age include: coronary heart disease, stroke, cancer, dementia, osteoporosis and musculoskeletal disorders.

It is for these and related reasons that the Institute of Medicine's National Research Agenda on Aging emphasizes the need to prevent the morbid sequel of aging and enhance positive health in the elderly to investigate the possibility of slowing biological aging.

In Ayurvedic classical literature, human body is considered as combination of earth, water, fire, air and space and they make not just the physical composition but also the mind and the spirit. That is, the body as a whole includes mind, soul, behaviour and consciousness of an individual where the environment also plays a major contribution in making of a person. - Charaka Sharir 6/4 Whereas in modern anatomy human body is made up of systems, tissues and cells from gross to subtle level.

According to Charaka, the combination of Chetana (life element) and Panchmahabhuta vikara is called Sharir and same is referred as Sthula Sharir. Sukshma Sharir is habitat of Jeewatma and Jeewatma resides in it. Sukshma Sharir is a group of 18 elements. Pertinently Ahankaara, mana, ten Indriyas and Tanmatras are the most important. Conjugation of Aatma possesed within Sukshma Sharir is addressed as 'linga Sharir'. Aatma with the linga Sharir holds and supports the whole body.

Aatma with the Sukshma Sharir provides Chetana (life element) to the Sthula sharir. The body is combination of Sharir, Indriya, Satva, Aatma. If one or more of these components are imbalanced or unconnected it can cause negative effect, such as disease. Charaka Samhita states that Satva or mind, Aatma or soul and Sharira or body are just like the legs of tripod, on which the world rests.

Consciousness in living body is represented by "invisible" energy field. In any diseases causing aging treatment at level of Pranamaya kosha (subtle body, Chakra) is of the most importance. Human energy field (Aura, Chakra) is surrounded by each energy field which is again surrounded by universal energy field.

A continuous exchange take place between the environment and the human body which is responsible for health and well being of human body. The methods and ways to the phenomena studied in bioenergetics. Clearing, balancing and energing the subtle body in all diseases is of equal importance as treatment at physical level. Energy (Chakra) healing is an important component of the treatment of cancer as bioenergetic medicine. The function of the emotion and mind even spiritual life.

Epigenetics is a new science and Ayurveda has been

around 5000 years. According to both conclusions are similar. As per the epigenetic research traditional ancient knowledge that diet, lifestyle and mindfulness can all be used to fight disease and promote health. Epigenetics which is literally our lifestyle controls us beyond genetics is a new field of biology that is exploring the impact of the environment on cellular behaviour.

During the past many years, various studies have been conducted on the physiological, psychological, and behavioral changes that aggravates the aging process. In every system decline in function with advancing age have been noted in virtually every system of the body. These include such clinically relevant domains as blood pressure, bone density, muscle mass, immune function, hearing, vision, renal function, glucose tolerance, pulmonary function, endocrine activity, and sympathetic nervous system activity.

Scientists have developed and validated the concept of "allostatic load" to describe and quantify the total wear and tear on the body's different systems due to repeated adaptation to various causes which induces stress. The effect of this load has been found to predict decrease in cognitive and physical functioning, the incidence of cardiovascular disease, and mortality in older adults.

The outcome of this has been explained to consist of two categories of biomarkers: (1) primary mediators—substances the body releases in response to stress such as nor epinephrine, epinephrine, cortisol, and de hydroepiandrosterone sulfate (DHEA-S) and (2) secondary meditator's resulting from the actions of primary mediators. Elevated systolic and diastolic blood pressures, cholesterol levels, glycated hemoglobin levels, and waist-to-hip ratio are few conditions involved. The changes with age in these physiological systems generally predispose to risk for disease, disability and mortality.

Neuro endocrine and immune systems are two major systems where changes have been reported because of regular wear and tear over the years. Reductions in T cell number and function, activation and proliferation of B cells and lower production of specific antibody have been found in various studies related to aging.

The major neuroendocrine changes with aging include: (a) declines in levels of the adrenal hormones - dehydroepian-drosterone and DHEA-sulfate (DHEAS), androstenedione, and progesterone, (b) decreased gonadal hormones, testosterone and estrogen, (c) decreased growth function hormones, growth hormone (GH) and insulin-like growth factor-1 (IGF-1), (d) changes in calcium metabolism hormones - decreased calcitonin and vitamin D and increased parathyroid hormone, (e) higher basal levels of hypothalamic-pituitary–adrenal (HPA) axis hormones - notably ACTH and cortisol.

Because of reductions in immune structure and function, accumulating evidence demonstrates increases in pro-inflammatory cytokines with aging. Ultimately these chemical mediators enhance inflammatory responses. It has been shown by substantial data that there is increase in the pro inflammatory cytokine & IL-6 level. This in turn induces products of the acute phase proteins, fibrinogen and C-reactive protein (CRP).

Ayurveda is the world's oldest and richest system of natural medicine, having its heritage in the ancient Vedic civilization of India. This science has been recognized by the World Health Organization as a best system of natural medicine with a detailed scientific literature consisting of classical medical texts, an oral tradition of knowledge, written texts, a comprehensive material medica, and a wide breadth of clinical procedures for prevention and treatment of acute and chronic diseases, as well as slowing the aging process.

"Ayus" in Sanskrit means life or lifespan. "Veda" means knowledge. The Ayurvedic tradition of knowledge and practice with its classical literature has been described as total knowledge of health and longevity.

Over the past 50 years, a systematic investigation and restoration of the original texts and practical applications of Ayurveda in light of modern scientific principles has been spearheaded in collaboration with leading physicians, scientists and Vedic scholars. Remarkably precise correlations between human neurophysiological structures and function and the aspects of the Ayurveda have been reported.

The mind approach of Ayurveda include various meditation programs to reduce psychosocial stress and optimize neurophysiological effects on mental, physical and social health. The physiological approach of Ayurveda includes herbal preparations or supplements for dissolution of physiological imbalances associated with the declines of aging, acute and chronic disorders. Other strategies are physiological purification and behavioural recommendations. The environmental approach takes advantage of the effects of the near environment (Vedic architecture) and distant environment (Vedic astrology) on health. Finally, there are technologies for reducing socio-environmental stress and enhancing public health.

Concept of Achar Rasayan in Ayurveda

The concept of psychological healing is a traditional meditation practice that has its origin in the ancient Vedic tradition of India. In past years, this technique has been extensively studied for its effects on mental, physical and behavioural health. Several clinical conditions and diseases which commonly afflict the aged have been studied with this practice. Orem-Johnson investigated the health insurance records of more than 2000 people practicing the meditation program over five years.

The outcome showed significantly less health care utilization by the meditation practitioners for all 11 major disease categories including heart disease and cancer when compared to other groups of similar age, gender, profession, and insurance terms. These findings were corroborated in Quebec, Canada by Herron et al who assessed healthcare utilization records of 679 Canadians for three years before and three years after learning meditation compared to normative data over the same period. The results showed that physician's payments for the experimental period during the pre-meditation baseline years were similar to the mean of participants of the same age and gender in the Quebec health insurance plan.

Epigenetics of Aging

There is certainly impact of environmental changes in the process of aging. The scientific studies done in this area has gathered a good data which is revealing the impact of DNA methylation aspects of aging. Till date the most significant discovery is the specificity by which the methylation status of some cytosine-guanine dinucleotides changes with age. Most of the changes to DNA methylation state were known to occur with age, it is nevertheless a surprise to behold the remarkable precision of this change and that it can be used itself as a measuring stick of biological age.

Because of this, many surprises have been revealed, including the uniformity of age from diverse tissues of a body, influences of internal and external factors on aging, and the distinctiveness of epigenetic aging from current understanding of aging. Very rapidly, the epigenetic clock has uncovered many novel aspects of aging and most excitingly it is challenging concepts of aging that we have long held to be correct or complete.

AYURVEDA AS BIOENERGETIC MEDICINE

Contemporary science tells us that the human organism is not just a physical structure made of molecules; but like everything else, is composed of energy fields. The human being is constantly changing, ebbing, and flowing, just like the sea. Scientists are learning to measure these subtle changes. The human energy field is the frontier for modern research, and the development of new diagnostic and treatment systems. This study is known as bioenergetic medicine.

The human being is always floating in a vast sea of life energy fields, thought fields, and bioplasmic forms. People have recognized this phenomenon in the past. It is being rediscovered. This is thus not a new phenomenon; but rather, a new observation, a growing awareness, a new perspective, and a renewed interest in studying the intricacies of the unknown.

HUMAN ENERGY FIELD (HEF)—SCIENTIFIC THEORIES

"A human being is a part of the whole, called by us the Universe, a part limited in time and space. The human being experiences himself, his thoughts and feelings as something separated from the rest- a kind of optical delusion of his consciousness. This type of delusion is a kind of prison for human being, restricting him to his personal desires and to affection for a few persons nearest to him. The human being must be to free from this prison by widening the circles of compassion to embrace all living creatures and the whole of nature in its beauty.

Ayurveda as bioenergetic medicine in aging in purview of Epigenetics

Recent advanced medicine focuses on the cutting-edge technologic breakthroughs such as the bionic pancreas or targeted gene therapy for treatment-resistant cancers. In contrast to this, an area of expanding interest within medicine is based on practices that are thousands of years old. Non pharmacological interventions are also known as mind-body medicine, these practices are as noted by the National Center for Complementary and Alternative Medicine, to "focus on the interactions among the brain, mind, body, and behavior, and on the powerful ways in which emotional, mental, social, spiritual, and behavioral factors can directly affect health" (nccam.nih.gov).

As per the 2007 National Health Interview Survey (NHIS), nearly 1 in 5 Americans reported using MBT a category encompassing meditation, yoga, tai chi, qigong, biofeedback, progressive muscle relaxation, guided imagery, hypnosis, and deep breathing exercises. Moreover, US adults spent more than $ 4.1 billion per year on MBT. Initial findings from the 2012 NHIS show a continuing increase in the use of yoga—8.4% of Americans practiced yoga in 2012, up from 6.1% in 2007.

Many such kind of techniques like yoga, tai chi, and qigong, originate from ancient spiritual traditions. All other MBTs, like hypnosis and progressive muscle relaxation, have more rich histories. Although MBTs vary, they share several key similarities, especially in health applications. Initially, MBTs involve regulation of the mind's attention processes to impact the body's physiology. Attention can be focused on a single object or mental process as in some forms of meditation, or on dynamic body postures as in tai chi or yoga.

Second, practice of MBTs usually precipitates parasympathetic activation, demonstrated by reduced blood pressure, heart rate, and oxygen consumption and increased vagal tone (heart rate variability). This physiologic effect, initially described as the relaxation response by Herbert Benson, is distinct from other parasympathetic-predominant states such as sleep and has been hypothesized to be a shared physiology among MBTs.

Finally, studies correlate MBTs with various neurobiological changes, including alterations in cortical thickness, default mode connectivity, and decreased insulin resistance. While the interplay between biological, psychological, biochemical, and genetic effects is not yet well understood, Taylor et al have hypothesized that the observed cortical, neuroendocrine, and molecular outcomes of regular MBT practice may be connected through an executive homeostatic network that links calming mental processes to the maintenance of homeostasis in physiological systems.

Because of their wide range of effects, MBTs have been studied in a variety of disease states. Evidence has shown the efficacy of MBTs in treating conditions such as cardiovascular disease, inflammatory disease, hypertension, irritable bowel syndrome, insomnia, chronic pain, depression, and posttraumatic stress disorder (PTSD). In aggregate, the effectiveness of MBT interventions is modest, and the specific mechanisms of action of MBT are not well understood.

Epigenetics and bioenergetic medicine studies :

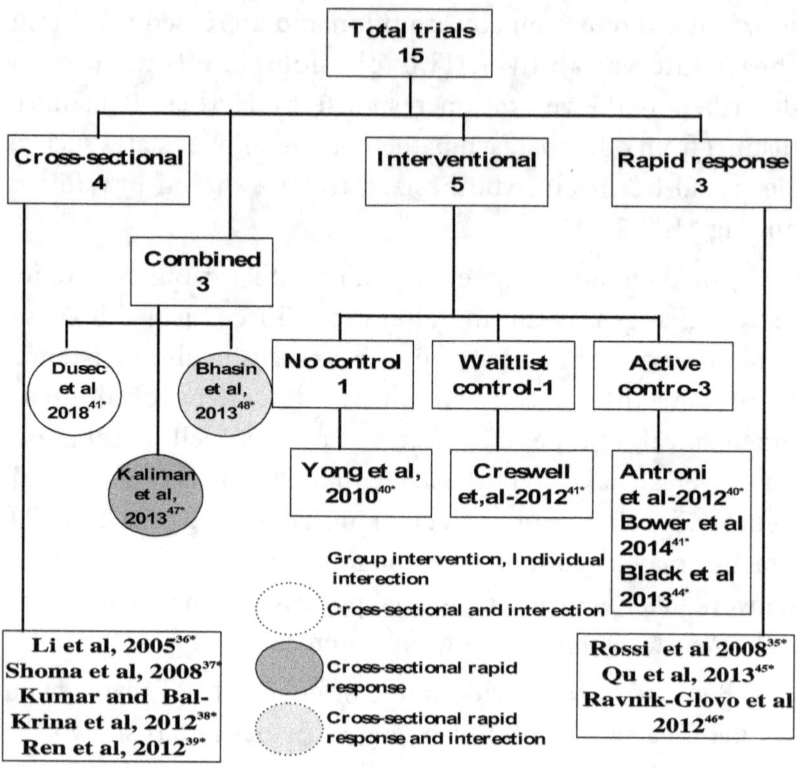

Conclusion

Human organism is not merely a physical structure which is made of molecules; but like everything else, is composed of energy fields._A continuous exchange take place between the environment and the human body which is responsible for health and well being of human body. The methods and approaches to the phenomena studied is bioenergetics. Clearing, balancing and energing the subtle body in all diseases is of equal importance as treatment at physical level. Energy (Chakra) healing is an important component of the treatment of any disease including aging as bioenergetic medicine.

The function of the emotion and mind even spiritual life. Many scientific studies have concluded with the explanation of effect of non pharmacological interventions in aging in purview of epigenetics. Treatment at level of Pranamayakosha (subtle body, Chakra) is of the most importance in reducing aging caused by any disease.

References:

- The Human Energy Field in Relation to Science, Consciousness, and Health By Gloria Alvino http:// arungowri.com/research/alvino01.pdf (http://arungowri.com/research/alvino01.pdf)
- Pooja Sabharwal, Rima Dada and Chetan Prakash. 2018. "Cancer and epigenetics interrelationship in prevention and cure", International Journal of Development Research, 8, (08), 22163-22168.
- The Corsini Encyclopaedia of psychology and Behavioral Science, Volume 4, Edited by W. Edward Craighead, Charles B. Nemeroff.
- Epigenetics of Aging and Longevity, Volume 4 in Translational Epigenetics, Book. 2018, Edited by Alexey Moskelev and Alexander M. Vaiserman.
- http://www.ozarkresearch.org/site/epigenetics.html.
- *Epigenetics – What Ayurveda Already Knows By Gwen Diaz.*www.ayurvedacollege.com
- Hands of Light: A guide to healing through the human energy field, by Barbara Ann Brennan.
- The Human Energy Field in Relation to Science, Consciousness, and Health By Gloria Alvino
- Functional Genomics in the Study of Mind-Body Therapieswww.ncbi.nlm.nih.gov pmc articles PMC 4295747

- Functional Genomics in the Study of Mind-Body Therapies by Halsey Niles et al.

- Masoro, E, Anstad, S and Rowe, J, *Handbook of the biology of aging.* 6th ed. 2006, New York: Academic Press.

- McEwen, B and Seeman, T, Protective and damaging effects of mediators of stress; elaborating and testing the concepts of allostasis and allostatic load. *Ann N Y Acad Sci*, 1999; (896): 30-47.

- Gruenewald, T and Kemeny, M, *Aging and Health: Psychoneuroimmunological processes*, in *The Handbook of Health Psychology and Aging*, C. Aldwin, C. Park, and A. Spiro, Editors. 2007, Guilford Press: New York, NY. p. 97-118.

- Seeman, TE, McEwen, BS, Rowe, JW and Singer, BH, Allostatic load as a marker of cumulative biological risk: Mac Arthur studies of successful aging. *Proceedings of the National Academy of Sciences U S A*, 2001; 98(8): 4770-5.

- Wan, H, Sengupta, M, Velkoff, V and De Barros, K, *65+ in the United States: 2005*, in *Current Population Reports*, U.C. Bureau, Editor. 2005, US Government Printing Office: Washington, DC.

- US Department of Health and Human Services. *Administration for Community Living.* 2014; Available from: https://aoa.acl.gov/Aging_Statistics/Index.aspx.

- Institute of Medicine (U.S.) and Lonergan, E, *extending life, enhancing life: a national research agenda on aging.* 1991, National Academy Press: Washington, D.C.

- Charak. Chapter 6, Shlok No.4. In: Charaka Samhita. Reprint-2012. New Delhi, Delhi: Chaukhamba Sanskrit

Sansthan, 2012; 787. Vidhyotini Hindi Commentary by Kashinath Shastri.

- Dilip KV. Section-3. In: Clinical Yoga & Ayurveda. 2011th ed. Delhi, Delhi: Chaukhamba Sanskrit Sansthanthan, 2011; 107–8.

- Chandra RBS. Chapter no.5. In: Gheranda Samhita. 2011th ed. Varanasi, U.P.: Chaukhamba Vidhyabhawann, 2011; 80–7.

- Trivedi Kshemkaran Das. Kand-10, Shlok-31. In: Athervaveda. 2012th ed. Delhi, Delhi: Arya Prakaashan, 2012; 236.

- Sabharwal Pooja. Discovery of the existence of human energy field (aura). unique journal of ayurvedic and herbal medicine, 2015 Mar 2; 62–3.

- Swerdlow RH. Bioenergetic medicine. British Journal of Pharmacology, 2014; 171(8): 1854–69.

- Introduction to Bioenergetic Medicine [Internet]. Holistic Health Alternatives. [cited 2018 Apr 14]. Available from: http://drdawn.net/learning-center/articles/introduction-to-bioenergetic-medicine/.

- Susruta. Sharir Sthan, Chapter no.4, Shlok no.3. In: Susruta Samhita. Reprint-2014. New Delhi, Delhi: Chaukhamba Publication, 2014; 14. Hindi Commentary by Kaviraj Ambika Dutta Shastri.

- Sabharwal pooja. Effect of intervrntion of Ayurveda & practical implementation of shadchakras an indigenous approch as co- therpy with chemotherapy & radiotherpy for physical & mental well being of cancer patient. Journal of ayurved A., Oct-dec 2008; 2: 28–33.

- Charak. Chapter 6, Shlok No.4. In: Charaka Samhita. Reprint-2012. New Delhi, Delhi: Chaukhamba Sanskrit

Sansthan, 2012; 787. Vidhyotini Hindi Commentary by Kashinath Shastri.

- Charaka. Sutra Sthan, Chapter no.1, Shlok no. 42. In: Charaka Samhita. Reprint-2012. New Delhi, Delhi: Chaukhamba Sanskrit Sansthan, 2012; 14. Vidhyotini Hindi Commentary by Kashinath Shastri.

- Charaka. Sutra Sthan, Chapter no.1, Shlok no. 46. In: Charaka Samhita. Reprint-2012. New Delhi, Delhi: Chaukhamba Sanskrit Sansthan, 2012; 18. Vidhyotini Hindi Commentary by Kashinath Shastri.

- Kamath nagraj. kriyatmakaanvrshana of shad chakaras. Unique journal of ayurvedic and herbal medicine, 2013 Mar 1; 34–6.

- Sabharwal pooja. Spiritual healing for cancer through chakras. In: Spiritual healing for cancer through chakras. 1st ed. Varanasi, U.P.: Chaukhamba Orientalia, 2009;1-14.

- Susruta. sutra sthana chapter 15, shlok no. 48, page no. 84. reprint-2014. Vol. 1. new delhi, delhi: chaukhambha publication; 2014. Ayurveda tattva sandipikahindi commentary by kavirajambikadutta shastri.

- Brian G Dias & Kerry J Ressler Parental olfactory experience influences behavior and neural structure in subsequent generations Nature Neuroscience, 2014; 17: 89–96.

- Beil, Laura (Winter 2008). "Medicine's New Epicenter? Epigenetics: New field of epigenetics may hold the secret to flipping cancer's "off" switch.". CURE (Cancer Updates, Research and Education).

- Bird, Adrian Perceptions of epigenetics Nature, 2007; 447(7143): 396-398.

- Gottlieb G "Epigenetic systems view of human development". Developmental Psychology, 27(1): 33–34.

- Aguilera, O., FernŒEndez, A. F., MuÛoz, A., & Fraga, M. F. (2010). Epigenetics and environment: A complex relationship. Journal of Applied [Manoj Jagtap et al: Enlightning Epigenetics Through Ayurveda And it's Role In Future] 294 www.ijaar.in VOL II ISSUE III SEP-OCT 2015 Physiology, 109: 243-251. Retrieved July 24, 2012, fromhttp://jap.physiology.org/content/109/1/243.full.pdf (PDF - 582 KB).

- Sinclair, K. D., Allegrucci, C., Singh, R., Gardner, D. S., Sebastian, S., Bispham, J., et al. (2007). DNA methylation, insulin resistance, and blood pressure in offspring determined by maternal periconceptional B vitamin and methionine status. Proceedings of the National Academy of Sciences, 104: 19351-19356.

- O'Connor, Anahad (11 March 2008). "The Claim: Identical Twins Have Identical DNA" New York Times. Retrieved 2 May 2010.

- Priya vrat Sharma Sushrut Samhita sharirsthana 5/3 Chaukhambha Visvabharati pg.170.

- Priya vrat Sharma Sushrut Samhita shaarirsthan 2/33 Chaukhambha Visvabharati pg.134.

- Y.G. Joshi Charak Samhita with Chakrapani commentary 4/32 Vaidyamitra Publication pg. 683.

- Prof. K.R. Srikantha Murty Astang Sangraha of Vagbhata 2/36 Chaukhambha Orientalia pg. 29.

- Manolio TA, Collins FS, Cox NJ, Goldstein DB, Hindorff LA, Hunter DJ, et al. Find- ing the missing heritability of complex diseases. Nature, 2009; 461: 747–53.

- Maher B. Personal genomes: the case of the missing heritability. Nature, 2008; 456: 18–21.

- Rakyan VK, Down TA, Balding DJ, Beck S. Epigenome-wide association studies for common human diseases. Nat Rev Genet, 2011; 12: 529–41.

- Chaturvedi MM, Sung B, Yadav VR, Kannappan R, Aggarwal BB. NF- kappa B addiction and its role in cancer: one size does not fit all'. Oncogene, 2011; 30: 1615–30.

- Messinaand M, Hilakivi-Clarke L. Early intake appears to be the key to the proposed protective effects of soy intake against breast cancer. Nutr Cancer, 2009; 61: 792–8.

- Shu XO, Zheng Y, Cai H, Gu K, Chen Z, Zheng W, et al. Soy food intake and breast cancer survival. JAMA, 2009; 302: 2437–43.

- Tennant DA, Duran RV, Gottlieb E. Targeting metabolic transformation for cancer therapy. Nat Rev Cancer, 2010; 10: 267–77.

- Boffetta P, Couto E, Wichmann J, Ferrari P, Trichopoulos D, Bueno-de- Mesquita HB, et al. Fruit and vegetable intake and overall cancer risk in the European Prospective Investigation into Cancer and Nutrition (EPIC). J Natl Cancer Inst, 2010; 102: 529–37.

- Binghamand S, Riboli E. Diet and cancer – the European prospective investi- gation into cancer and nutrition. Nat Rev Cancer, 2004; 4: 206–15.

- Huang J, Plass C, Gerhauser C. Cancer chemoprevention by targeting the epigenome. Curr Drug Targets, 2011; 12: 1925–56.

- 2010; 80: 1816–32. vel Szic KS, Ndlovu MN, Haegeman G, Vanden Berghe W. Nature or nurture: let food be your epigenetic medicine in chronic inflammatory disorders. Biochem Pharmacol.

- Pooja S, Bibhuprasad N, Akanksha S. Pranic Healing: A Stress Buster For Cancer Patients. International Journal of Advanced Research, 2019; 7(1): 380–4.

- Leeand BM, Mahadevan LC. Stability of histone modifications across mam- malian genomes: implications for epigenetic' marking. J Cell Biochem, 2009; 108: 22–34.

- Vanden Berghe W, Ndlovu MN, Hoya-Arias R, Dijsselbloem N, Gerlo.

- S, Haegeman G. Keeping up NF-kappaB appearances: epigenetic control of immunity or inflammation-triggered epigenetics. Biochem Pharmacol.

●

9 Ayurinformatics & Epigenetics

Ayur-informatics is a branch of science which deals with the application of bioinformatics to the Ayurvedic medication. Bioinformatics is merging of Biology and Computers. Bioinformatics is the field of science in which biology, computer science, and information technology unite into a single branch. It is the science of managing and analyzing biological data by utilizing advanced computing techniques. The ultimate goal of bioinformatics is to enable the discovery of new biological insights as well as to create a global perspective from which unifying principles in biology can be applied.

Computers & Bioinformatics:

Bioinformatics is the discipline in which computer-assisted data management helps to gather, store, analyze, and integrate biological and genetic information. This information is further represented efficiently. Databases of gene and protein sequence and structure/function information databases are produced by using the science of bioinformatics. New sequences, new structures or protein/gene function that are discovered are searched & then compared against already gathered data.

In bioinformatics analysis and interpretation of various types of biological data including nucleotide and amino acid sequences, protein domains, and protein structures is done. Development of new algorithms and statistics from which the biological information is assessed such as relationships among members of large data sets is done. DNA Chips, Micro Array, and Gene expression data to be analyzed are few examples of biological data for bioinformatics. Examples of Proteins are Proteome of an Organism, 2D Structure & 3D Structure.

Ayur-informatics

It is an attempt to provide a scientific platform to the traditional Indian medications. There has been an increase in demand for the phytopharmaceutical products of Ayurveda in contemporary medicine world because of the fact that the allopathic drugs have more side effects.

Ayur informatics in Oncology treatment

With the advancement of new technologies, the molecular biology of cancer development as well as apoptotic pathways are becoming clear to us. Mitochondria play an important role in the internal 'intrinsic' apoptotic pathway (Dixon et al. 2007). Many scientists have shown interest in targeting the proteins involved in mitochondrial apoptotic pathway to develop new anticancer drugs. By applying the modern drug designing technologies and bioinformatics to the traditional Ayurveda it can proved to be a boon to the Medical Science. (International Journal of Bioscience, Biochemistry and Bioinformatics, Vol. 1, No. 1, May 2011).

Examples of Ayurinformatics

There are various examples of Ayurinformatics, One of them is Bronchial carcinoma which is the world's most common type of cancer associated with the mutations of ras, src, and myc genes and tumor suppressor proteins p53 and BRCA1 along with the epidermal growth factor receptors (EGFR). After generating 3D structures of these proteins by using homology modelling. Medicinal herbs and plants were selected on the basis of their properties of their active compounds. Chemical structures of the active components of these herbs were drawn using chem. sketch, combined and converted to*.pdb.

The proteins were successfully in silico docked with the combination of active components. Few studies suggest that p53 and H-ras mutations are frequent and apparently independent genetic alterations which play different roles in the pathogenesis, progression and prognosis of non small cell lung cancer. The functions of BRCA1in DNA damage response give a reasonable molecular explanation for its role as a tumor suppressor.

Ayurvedic medications of Bronchial carcinoma

Berberine is an isoquinoline alkaloid, It is isolated from root of Burberis vulgaris Berberine arrests cancer cell cycle in G1 phase and induces apoptosis. It exhibits immunoenhancing, antioxidant and anti- inflammatory properties. Similarly Curcumin has impressive medicinal qualities.

In a study conducted by the United States National Cancer Institute, the scientists have noted the role of turmeric (Curcumin), an ingredient in common Indian curry spice for prevention of cancer. Curcumin is present in Curcumin longa (turmeric). Curcumin arrests the cancer cells proliferation in G2/S phase and induces apoptosis Daidzein is an isoflavone, which is a hormone-like substance found in soybeans.

After genistein, Daidzein is the second most plentiful isoflavone in soy. It inhibits the growth of cancer by taking the place of estrogen on receptors in cancerous cells that actually need estrogen to grow. When Homology Modelling was done for the proteins RAS, MYC, SRC, BRCA1, P53 and

EGFR using Modeller9v7, for the amino acid sequence of each protein was retrieved from NCBI's database and advance modeling was used (taking three templates for each protein) for modeling the structures.

By doing so, the best model is docked with suitable ligand. Lingands used for each protein are as follows:

- RAS: Limonene, Berberine and Curcumin combination.

- BRCA1: Podophyllotoxin, D-Limonene and Sulforaphane combination.

- P53:   Vindoline, Berberine and Curcumin combination

- EGFR: Oleanolic Acid, Ursolic Acid and Emodin combination.

It is found out that the ligands (combination of active compounds) docks with the corresponding proteins. The ligand found to bind the protein in an effective manner and this can be effective in treating bronchial carcinoma. As this study was an in-silico work, to establish its efficacy the compound combinations has to go to clinical trials.

In order to discover novel ligands for receptors of known structure in silico molecular docking is one of the most power-ful and useful techniques. It has a major role in structure-based drug designing (Brooijmans et al. 2003). Few studies like for finding Ayurvedic remediation for Ebola hemorrhagic fever (Bagchi et al. 2009) by homology modeling with in silico docking and medication for Alzheimer's disease (Gore et al. 2010) were previously reported. An in silico molecular docking was done to investigate whether the active compounds from ginger could bind to NADH oxido reductase enzyme as ligands is another eample of such study. Active Compounds from ginger as

Inducers of Mitochondrial Apoptotic Pathway: An in Silico Prediction the enzyme NADH dehydrogenase can be an important target for natural drugs in this respect. Active compounds of ginger (Zingiber officinale Roscoe) namely gingerol, paradol, shogaol and zingerone were selected as ginger is known to have anti-cancer properties.

In one in silico study a three-dimensional model of the human NADH dehydrogenase was developed and docked with gingerol, paradol, shogaol and zingerone. Successful docking was done for all of them. The most potent for drug development among the active components of ginger was isolated with the successful docking of these natural compounds with the enzyme as they showed that these two compounds, namely 6-gingerol and 10-gingerol, formed covalent bonds with the enzyme are potential inducers of the apoptotic pathway and thus important in chemotherapeutic drug development. Chemical structures of [6]-gingerol, [8]-gingerol, [10]-gingerol, [6]-shogaol, [6]-paradol and zingerone were downloaded from KEGG (Kanehisa and Goto 2000) chemical database (http://www.genome.jp/kegg/) and 3D rendering were done by ACD/Chem Sketch (Freeware. The 3D rendered structures were saved as *.mol file and converted to *.pdb file using ArgusLab 4.0.1 (Thompson 2004) downloaded from http://www.arguslab.com. These structures were used as ligands for docking with the 3D modeled NADH dehydrogenase.

Another example is blocking the translation pathway of fumarate hydratase mutation gene by rnai technique and establishing an ayurvedic remedy for uterine fibroids . In this study fumarate hydratase precursor (mutation) protein of Homo sapiens was taken. Homology modeling studies were done and 3D structure of FH protein was modelled. Ayurvedic herbs Aloe vera, Commiphora mukul, Asparagus racemosa and Saraca indica's active components were selected, combined & docked with Fumarate hydratase mutation protein. The docking proves that the combination is effective in curing uterine fibroids. The Fumarate Hydratase mutation protein, human FH was retrieved from Uni Prot database (accession number P07954) for this work. Homology modeling studies were done using modeler 9v7 software using templates (homologous proteins in the RCSB's pdb database). The chemical structure of aloe-emodin, guggul-sterone, shatavarin and 17-ketosterol were drawn using ACD/ Chemsketch software. The structures of aloeemodin, guggul-sterone, shatavarin and 17 ketosterol were merged as one structure (proposed treatment). This combination is converted to 3d which was converted to *.pdb. There are many other examples like a computational epigenetics research group at the Max Planck Institute for Informatics in Saarbr¤ucken is using software programs to rummage through the genomes of cancer patients in search for suspicious methylation patterns. These patterns in clinical diagnosis as biomarkers and combined with ingenious algorithms were used and statistical processes, researchers have developed an epigenetic bio-marker for malignant glioblastoma.

Ayurinformatics and epigenetics

The epigenetic science is the new field of discussion among researchers. Scientists are constantly doing experiments on biochemical modifications beyond the actual DNA strand to lead to huge progress in the understanding of the regulation of gene activity in near future. Two scientists Thomas Lengauer and Christoph Bock from the Max Planck Institute for Informatics in Saarbr¤ucken have demonstrated by their work that how epigenetics research is applicable in medical application. The human body which consists of a scarcely conceivable 10 to 100 billion cells, out of these few diseased cells causes cancer. Only minor damage in the DNA as a result of exposure to UV light or tobacco smoke can switch off a cell's natural growth limits: the cell then starts to divide uncontrollably and, in the very bad condition, overgrow healthy tissue in the form of tumors, which eventually destroy vital organs.

Earlier it was believed that changes in the DNA itself play a crucial role in the emergence of cancer. but it is now clear that the modification of the DNA strand also has an important role to play, as a cell's genetic material is modified by a large number of chemical attachments. DNA methylation and histone modification play a central role in gene regulation: small hydrocarbon attachments thus decide whether a gene is "active" or "silenced", namely whether it can be read off or not. The defects in DNA methylation result in altered gene activity in the cell which can contribute to tumor formation. The methylation patterns of tumor cells differ clearly from those of healthy tissue cells. This is the area where scientists are targeting. The scientists are working through vast collections of genetic data for suspicious methylation patterns using software programs they develop themselves. In very specific types of cancer, these patterns arise so they can be use in clinical diagnosis as biomarkers, also as indicators for the corresponding form of the disease," says Thomas Lengauer. The scientists rely on close cooperation with hospitals and biotechnology laboratories for their work. The tissue samples from cancer patients a were processed in the laboratory and the genetic material they contain was cut into numerous small snippets. The solution was then processed using microarrays (DNA chips) or using new-generation sequencing processes. A kind of map of the epigenome was generated which comprises all of the biochemical markings layered on top the actual DNA sequence, as explained by Thomas Lengauer. And all of this effort is proving worth while. There is a report that scientists are working in collaboration with the UniversitŠtsklinikum Bonn. The scientists in SaarbrŸcken also developed an epigenetic biomarker for malignant glioblastoma, which is the most common form of malignant brain tumor. Christoph Bock, who leads a research group at the Research Center for Molecular Medicine in Vienna explains that "Chemotherapy is only effective in around one quarter of affected patients". "In these cancer patients, a particular gene called MGMT is methylated, that is silenced. When it is in its active state, this gene controls a repair mechanism in the cancer cells. In patients where active MGMT is present, the DNA damage arising during chemotherapy, which causes diseased cells to die, would be reversed and the treatment fails." With the knowledge of the new biomarker, the scientists, doctors can now identify in advance of treatment for those patients for whom debilitating chemotherapy is actually worthwhile.

The researchers recent success has also opened up completely new paths in clinical cancer diagnosis. In one of the major international project headed by Manel Esteller from the Bellvitge Biomedical Research Institute in Barcelona, Spain, over 1,600 human tissue samples were analyzed. Then the methylation pattern was sampled at around 1,500 characteristic places in each analyzed genome and the resulting data analyzed by computer at the MPI in SaarbrŸcken. The results of the analysis are very promising. Although in around 25 percent of cases, this search is not that successful. As cancer cells frequently degenerate outside their original tissue, without knowing the origin of the primary tumor, it is almost impossible to establish what kind of cancer is involved and this, in turn, significantly reduces the patient's chances of a successful cure. Recently, the potential offered by epigenome mapping has also been recognized at an international level. There are many major projects which are being coordinated under the aegis of the International Epigenome Consortium (IHEC). The main aim is to completely map the epigenomes of at least 1,000 biologically and medically significant cell types and cell states. The individual projects within the IHEC focus on different issues. In the united states institutes are aiming to create reference profiles for as many healthy human cell types as possible, the EU-funded BLUEPRINT project is focusing on the cells of the blood and immune system Thomas Lengauer regards epigenome analysis as playing a important role in the attainment of rapid progress in cancer diagnosis in the coming days, he is keen with regard to the development of new drugs. Many scientists have mentioned about the potential of future drugs that can repair defects in the epigenome of diseased cells. Such targeted interventions involve significant risks, not least because little or nothing much is known about the highly-complex gene regulation mechanisms being manipulated here."

- https://www.ncbi.nlm.nih.gov/Class/MLACourse/Modules/MolBioReview/bioinformatics.html
- https://alttox.org/mapp/emerging-technologies/omics-bioinformatics-computational-biology/
- https://www.authorstream.com/Presentation/jyotirath-1560238-introduction-bioinformatics/
- https://www.nature.com/articles/nbt1000_it31
- https://umccc.org.au/all-movies-biryk/e5d64b-bioin-formatics-pdf-drive
- https://www.researchgate.net/publication/269799944

Ayur-Informatics_Establishing_an Ayurvedic Remedy for_Bronchial_Carcinoma

- https://www.ijbs.com/v05p0020.htm
- http://www.vitaminstuff.com/daidzein.html
- https://pdfs.semanticscholar.org/16bc/5c7c0e9b d42623997c72b760adef5a0592ea.pdf
- https://www.researchgate.net/publication/47530691 Ayur-informatics_Establishing_an_in-silico-ayurvedic medication for Alzheimer's_disease
- https://www.researchgate.net/publication/50250712 Structure modeling_of_novel_DNA glycosylase enzyme_from oral_pathogen_Streptococcus sanguinis
- https://www.researchgate.net/publication/296639039 Active_Compounds_from Ginger_as Inducers of Mitochondrial Apoptotic Pathway An in Silico Prediction
- https://bipublication.com/files/phv1i120104.pdf
- https://scitechdaily.com/researchers-use-bioinformatics-and-epigenetics-to-aid-cancer-research/
- https://www.mpg.de/5053760/bioinformatics epigenetics
- https://www.ncbi.nlm.nih.gov/pmc/articles PMC1421942

10 $~$ **F**uture **Perspective**

An individual is result of present, past and his ancestral environment which is ultimate result of various changes on the epigenome of the individual. Various scientific studies have come with the opinion of involvement of epigenetic changes which has effect on various systems of the human body.

Scientific knowledge about changes caused to epigenome of the human body are possible to understand. As there is complex mechanism involved for the alternations occurring on epigenome because of the lifestyle & environment. Taking the advantage of this understanding it is very much possible to reverse the changes of epigenome with intervention of pharmacological and non pharmacological interventions in various diseases.

As mentioned in earlier chapters mainly two processes are involved in epigemone changes which are hyper/hypo methylation and histone modifications. Scientists are targeting mainly on these two factors after interventions of dietary and lifestyle changes.

Craig Venter a pioneer genomic researcher has done a rigorous research in this field. He has declared in a conference that "Human biology is actually far more complicated than we imagine. Our genes are responsible for our fate this is what we have heard till date. But it is not true, genes expression is responsible for the changes. And the expression of the genes is actually outcome of life style, diet and environment of the individual and his/her ancestors.

Genetic composition actually gives us information about our basic constitution and the vulnerability of the diseases. The actual onset of the disease still depends upon the diet, lifestyle and environment of the individual.

Epigenetics is a new science, but traditional Indian medicine which is old age science both have same conclusion. Now a day's epigenetic research has confirmed that intervention of traditional India medicine has impact in reversal of disease with the epigenetic background.

Genetic expression changes due to multiple factors change into mutations whatever we are doing, eating, listening has impact on genetic expression at very minute level.

Lifelong remodeling of our epigenome is possible. Fruits, vegetables, teas, spices, and medicinal herbs have components that can regulate multiple cancer and inflammatory pathways via epigenetics Drugs that target a single gene product are unlikely to be of use in preventing or treating cancer. Chronic dreadful diseases like cancers have long latency periods, safe and effective multi-functional treatments that act on entire networks in the body are required.

Bioactive components in food may prevent or treat metabolic diseases via epigenetics Curcumin, sulforaphane, diindolylmethane (DIM), Indol-3-carbinol (I3C), Phenethyliso-thiocyanate (PEITC), Epigallocatechin-3-gallate (EGCG), genistein, quercetin, resveratrol, ellagitannins, butyrate, organo-sulfur compounds, lycopene.

Epigenetics is a personlized medicine. The contemporary science is developing new drugs which target specific epigenetic components. It recognizes that diet, lifestyle and the environment can have epigenetic effects. The future therapy may include drugs with epigenetic targets: DNA-MT inhibitors, HDAC inhibitors, etc.

In Ayurvedic approach for each person treatments are person specific. There are certainly roles of body, mind, and spirit in maintaining health which have been recognized. In near future treatment for diseases may include changes in diet and/or lifestyle, as well as medicinal herbs and panchakarma therapies. Medications are chosen based on their unique characteristics (Rasa, Guna, Virya, Vipaka, and Prabhava) and the Prakriti and Vikriti of the person being treated.

A person is experiencing health or is susceptible to disease is determined by mind, body & spirit which are three pillars of health. Disease occurs due to imbalances in any of these three pillars. It is very well explained in charak samhita i.e "Every individual is different from another and hence should be considered as a different entitity. As many variations as there are in the universe, all are seen in human beings".

- https://1library.net/document/yr27jevz-cancer-and-epigenetics-interrelationship-in-prevention-and-cure.html
- https://www.academia.edu/36631048/Integrative_Ayurveda_Oncology_Where_We_Are_And_Way_Ahead

●

www.ingramcontent.com/pod-product-compliance
Lightning Source LLC
Chambersburg PA
CBHW070534160726
48003CB00004B/1777